THE 2–DAY SUPERFOOD CLEANSE

THE 2-DAY SUPERFOOD CLEANSE

A WEEKLY DETOX PROGRAM TO BOOST ENERGY, LOSE WEIGHT AND MAINTAIN OPTIMAL HEALTH

ROBIN WESTEN

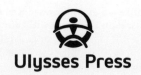

Ulysses Press

Published in the U.S. by:
Ulysses Press
P.O. Box 3440
Berkeley, CA 94703
www.ulyssespress.com

ISBN13: 978-1-61243-292-2
Library of Congress Control Number: 2013957322

Printed in the United States by United Graphic Inc.

Acquisitions Editor: Katherine Furman
Managing Editor: Claire Chun
Editor: Lauren Harrison
Proofreader: Elyce Berrigan-Dunlop
Index: Sayre Van Young
Front cover design: TG Design
Cover artwork: © Acambium64/shutterstock.com
Interior design and layout: what!design @ whatweb.com

10 9 8 7 6 5 4 3 2 1

Distributed by Publishers Group West

To my son, Gabriel Sky Westen, who shows me the way.

Table of Contents

Acknowledgments

Special thanks to editor-supreme, Katherine Furman, as well as to Ulysses Press and their amazing production and publicity teams. Also to my DUMBO hood, especially the gang at 68 Jay and Olympia, whose compassionate support helped to make this book possible. Gratitude is offered to Abhaya Yoga's superlative teachers and its heart-centered community, who join together on the journey of opening. Thanks to friends in Vermont who walk the wooded paths alongside me and help to grow ideas. Finally, deepest appreciation to my true soul match, Dr. Bebop, my husband and best friend–forever.

Introduction

It was tough to ignore the signs when nature urged me to make a new start. I looked in the mirror and suddenly saw myself as if for the first time – and it wasn't a pretty sight. My complexion was dull, eyes without sparkle; rather than standing tall and confident, my shoulders and neck turned inward and my muffin top could easily serve four. I can joke about it now, but back then it wasn't so funny. My energy was in a slump and any drive and creativity felt out of reach. At this crossroads I had a choice: to accept these conditions as an inevitable decline and continue existing without really experiencing the fullness of life, or to stop the wheel, reverse the process, and thrill once more to living.

The choice was obvious, but the solution wasn't so simple. There was no instant way to cleanse my body and spirit. One day of watching what I ate or what I thought or randomly paying attention to potential toxins in my environment didn't result in a permanent solution. In order to truly change, I realized I had to not only become conscious of toxic conditions but maintain the will to seek out a more purified state. I needed to exchange my random diet for one where I paid attention to when and what I consumed. I needed to replenish and nourish my body and brain, boost my energy level, help to cleanse toxins from my system, and hopefully lose weight in the process.

But I was realistic, too. There was no way I could manage to stay on a narrow cleansing path 24/7. I knew that any program I embarked on would have to give me plenty of leeway to socialize with friends and family in a relaxed way. I didn't want to have to worry about what I was eating when I was with them, and I didn't want to always be on guard when I was home alone and felt like indulging a bit. I tried strict programs before and they never worked. So, I wondered: "Was it possible to detox and cleanse *part-time* and still see results?"

I'm happy to report the answer is a resounding *YES!* The secret? Superfoods. These multitasking morsels supply the body and spirit with an abundance of vitamins, minerals, and protein while cleansing toxins from our organs and helping to promote weight loss by encouraging our digestive system to work at peak levels. Countless studies confirm superfoods have the potential to ward off disease, crank up energy, enliven mood, build muscle, diminish fat, and even increase longevity.

The Two-Day Superfood Cleanse is a real-life program that utilizes the power of hypernutrition coupled with the detoxing benefits of cleansing. Simply, all you need to do is devote *any* two days during the week to a 600-calorie Superfood Cleanse. The other days you can eat whatever you like. This is similar to the popular 5:2 diet, but instead of just reducing calories, you engage the heath factor by eating detoxing superfoods on your two cleanse days. And superfoods take away cravings, which means on low-calorie days you won't feel hungry or deprived. I've been following this program for two years and in the process I lost 15 pounds within the first six months (and kept it off), gained back my energy three-fold, and I feel more optimistic and committed to exploring the deeper well of my inner world than ever before.

On the following pages, you'll read about 35 superfoods, their physical, emotional, and mental benefits, and the ways in which they support both cleansing and weight loss. You'll also be given the calories in each of these amazing foods so you can keep track of where you are within the daily 600-calorie limit. If you're wondering which foods will personally benefit you the most, take the quiz on page 24 to find out.

In Chapter Two you'll get a historical, cultural, and medicinal look at fasting, cleansing, and dieting, as well as an explanation of the recent, wildly popular 5:2 approach. You'll learn why staying on a low-calorie diet for only two days a week works and why cleansing rather than arbitrary low-calorie fasting is the way to go in today's toxic world. But everyone is different, so take the quiz in this chapter on page 39 to "Discover Your Personality Secrets in Your Favorite Foods."

In the following chapter you'll be given the hands-on tools to maintain your Two-Day Superfood Cleanse, including calorie-counting tips, ways to understand nutritional content, how to keep track of portion size, instructions to prepare ingredients, tips for smart shopping, and information on supplements and juicing. "Are You Ready for the Two-Day Superfood Cleanse?" Take the quiz on page 59 to find out.

You'll not only learn about the most common setbacks to successful dieting, but in Chapter Four, readers are offered exercises to avoid these traps by strengthening willpower, firming commitment, and bolstering positive thinking. Take the "What Gives You a Winning Edge?" quiz on page 77 and discover your willpower quotient. Then read the custom-designed suggestions to help boost your personal resolve.

Chapter Five offers dozens of recipes for simple, low-calorie juices, salads, soups, and side dishes, all made with a concentration of superfoods. Each recipe is well under the 600-calorie limit and lists the calorie content so you can keep track of how many you've consumed during a cleanse day.

To go beyond calorie counting, Chapter Six explores concrete ways readers can embrace a physically and emotionally nontoxic and reduced-stress life, including directions on how to make a clean sweep of your environment, instructions for special cleansing yoga poses, simple guidelines for meditation, and deep-breathing practices, as well as descriptions of several additional techniques to help cleanse not only your body but your emotional world, too. Finally, take the "Rate Your Progress" quiz on page 133 and get a picture of your progress.

Once your body harnesses the power of cleansing and you drop those unwanted pounds, you'll achieve your maximum mental, emotional, and physical potential. Why wait? Begin today and experience what your body is *truly* craving – nutritional balance, weight loss, and ultimate wellness.

1

Superfoods for a Two–Day Clean Sweep

To keep the body in good health is a duty, otherwise we shall not be able to keep our mind strong and clear.
~ Buddha

Ask some conventional, doubting Thomas types about the power of superfoods and they might pass the plate. It's their loss. Numerous studies conducted for more than a decade confirm that these multitasking eatables pack a powerhouse of health–filled benefits. Superfoods optimize *all* our body's systems, helping it to function at full–blast and maximum capacity. They're megarich with essential nutrients, antioxidants, vitamins, minerals, essential fatty acids, and protein. Stacks of research show that if you choose these superfoods as the center of your diet, you can reduce the risk of chronic disease, raise your serotonin (the feel–good brain chemical) level, boost your immune system, fine-tune your metabolism, enhance your sexuality, bump up your brain power, and help yourself look and feel more vibrant. They can even prolong life. Simply put, if you eat more of these magnificent morsels, you'll be a whole lot healthier, happier, and stronger. Plus, when you make superfoods the center of your Two-Day Cleanse and support your body's optimal digestion, you'll also be thinner.

Despite the life-changing benefits of these foods, you don't have to travel far and wide, or even to an overpriced health food store to get your fill. Most are easy to find. They can usually be bought at your local farmer's market when seasonal fruits and vegetables are available or in the organic section of your neighborhood grocery store.

Whenever possible...
Go organic
Choose what's in season

A Fresh Start

There are very few of us who weren't raised eating fruits and vegetables sprayed with pesticides, meat pumped with antibiotics, and dairy enhanced with antibiotics, not to mention vitamin- and mineral-lacking, calorie-packed, ultraprocessed foods. But once you focus on eating superfoods, that's history; you can kiss your old eating habits, and your former out-of-shape body, good-bye. With the Two-Day Superfood Cleanse, you gain the opportunity to realign your physical systems, your mind, and your emotional world, and to rid each of built-up toxins. Since you'll get a boost in vitality from changing your diet, you'll see the world with a new set of sparkling eyes. You'll be given the gift of living your life with a clear sense of awareness and gratitude. You'll literally experience, through every pore in your body, a consistent flow of energy.

What's more, when you choose a Superfood Cleanse, you'll not only lose weight but keep your bones strong, muscles sinewy, and inner organs functioning at their peaks. Just think about your Superfood Cleanse as medicine that tastes totally yummy. Superfoods can come in the form of fruits, vegetables, seeds, and nuts. Take note that when you eat these nutrient- and protein-rich foods, they also help to fine-tune your digestive system and make your tummy feel full. The result? So long, cravings!

On the following pages you'll learn about the nutritional properties of superfoods and their caloric measurement. Choose among these foods during your two cleanse days while calculating calories and paying attention to portions, and you'll achieve long-term weight loss and remarkable wellness.

Here Are the Top Superfoods

Look no further than the list below to find delicious and ultranutritious foods. Always keep portion size in mind when consuming these delectable choices. Too much of a good thing can be a common trap for dieters.

Nuts

Those who consume nuts five times a week have about a 50 percent reduction in risk of heart attack according to the Loma Linda School of Public Health.

ALMONDS: Ranking high in vitamin E content (an essential vitamin that combines with oxygen and destroys free radicals), almonds have amazing anti-aging properties. For example, it was discovered that the flavonoids in almond skins work in synergy with the nut's vitamin E to reduce the risk of heart disease. These nuts also help to build strong bones and teeth thanks to their phosphorus content. They even provide healthy fats that can aid in weight loss. Fats help you absorb vitamins A, D, and of course, E, and they're vital for your nervous system. These fats raise good HDL cholesterol, lower bad LDL cholesterol, and protect against the buildup of plaque in your arteries. They also help prevent belly fat, according to research. What's more, with its riboflavin and L-carnitine (nutrients that boost brain activity) almonds may lower the risk of Alzheimer's disease.

5 WHOLE ALMONDS: 35 calories

BRAZIL NUTS: These crescent moon–shaped nuts are good for your heart because they contain monounsaturated fats that help to reduce levels of so-called bad cholesterol. But what makes them super extraordinary is their whopping selenium content. An extremely rich source of this mineral, just one Brazil nut a day can provide you with your entire recommended daily intake, according to research. Selenium protects the body from free radicals, and studies show that folks who eat a diet rich in this mineral are less likely to suffer from cancer compared to those with a poor intake. Note: Keep Brazil nuts in the fridge or freezer as they quickly spoil once shelled.

6 WHOLE BRAZIL NUTS: 137 calories

PINE NUTS: Rich in vitamin A and lutein, pine nuts not only support vision and contain heart-friendly monounsaturated fat, but they possess a sizable vitamin D content that helps build strong bones. Thanks to their abundance of vitamin C, pine nuts also elevate the body's immunity. Pine nuts contain pinolenic acid, which makes you feel fuller faster and thus aids in weight loss. Since they're a good source of iron, these nuts boost both our circulatory and nervous systems. And if you're feeling fatigued, eating a handful of pine nuts will lift you up. The reason? Plenty of protein and magnesium.

80 PINE NUTS: 95 calories

WALNUTS: Walnuts are rich sources of vitamins B and E, calcium, manganese, potassium, and protein. This superfood is considered to be nourishment for the brain because it improves your mind's function significantly. Walnuts also contain alpha–linolenic omega–3 fatty acids, which can curb food cravings and aid weight loss. The FDA recommends eating a handful of walnuts every day to lower LDL levels and to improve overall lipid profile. Walnuts are effective in preventing depression and anxiety and can also regulate blood sugar levels in people suffering from diabetes. As an added bonus, walnuts are powerful antioxidants and possess anti-inflammatory properties.

5 WHOLE WALNUTS WITH SKIN: 131 calories

Seeds

If you can look into the seeds of time, and say which grain will grow and which will not, speak then unto me.

~ William Shakespeare

BUCKWHEAT GROATS: Buckwheat groats are the hulled seeds of the buckwheat plant. This health bonanza has been cultivated for at least 1,000 years in China, Korea, and Japan, where it's often enjoyed in the form of buckwheat "soba" noodles. Buckwheat has more protein than rice, wheat, millet, or corn and is high in the essential amino acids lysine and arginine. Its relative proportions of amino acids make it one of the top cholesterol–lowering foods available. It also has the ability to reduce and stabilize our blood sugar and help tame hypertension. What's more, a study out of Madrid, Spain, determined that buckwheat contains high levels of probiotics, the helpful bacteria in our digestive system that works to keep our metabolism functioning at peak levels.

½ CUP BUCKWHEAT GROATS: 77 calories

CHIA SEEDS: Okay, stop laughing. You don't have to eat your Chia Pet, but you definitely should consider adding these morsels to your diet. The itty bitty black and white seeds are packed with omega-3 fatty acids, carbohydrates, protein, dietary fiber, antioxidants, and calcium. Since they have a sort of nutty flavor, chia seeds are easy to add to a variety of foods and drinks; and when they're mixed with water they create a gel that may act as an appetite suppressant. Along the same lines, chia seeds are currently being studied as a potential natural treatment for type-2 diabetes because of their ability to slow digestion.

2 TABLESPOONS CHIA SEEDS: 138 calories

CHOCOLATE: Wondering why chocolate is in the seed section? It's because the cocoa tree grows cocoa pods (the fruit) and inside the cocoa pod you find cocoa beans, which are actually seeds. It may be a bit confusing, but this much we know for sure: Chocolate is delicious and a surefire superfood. This sweet treat contains flavonoids, which act as antioxidants to protect the body from damage caused by free radicals, which can lead to heart disease, maybe even cancer. Flavonoids help relax blood pressure through the production of nitric oxide, and they also balance certain hormones in the body. Chocolate is also reported to improve digestion and stimulate the kidneys. It has been used to help people with anemia, kidney stones, and poor appetite. What's more, it lessens anxiety by producing the neurotransmitter serotonin thanks to the tryptophan in the chocolate. The best kind of chocolate is dark and minimally processed. On the downside, all chocolate contains approximately 6 milligrams (mg) of caffeine per ounce of chocolate, which is about the amount found in decaffeinated coffee. Although this is a lot less than what is found in a typical serving of soda or coffee, for those with specific heart conditions, such as palpitations or arrhythmia, chocolate may not be as beneficial. Note: Chocolate can be a bit addictive (as you might already know!).

1 OUNCE CHOCOLATE: 155 calories

FLAXSEEDS: This nutty–flavored seed provides heaps of nutrition, but only when it's ground. Studies have found that flaxseed can not only help to prevent heart disease but also offer protection against breast, cervical, and ovarian cancers. Flaxseed is fantastic in other ways: A 2010 study in the *Journal of Nutrition* reports that it may even help reduce belly fat. What gives flaxseed its punch? It contains both omega–3s and phytoestrogens called lignans. It turns out that flax has more of these plant compounds than any other food on the planet. Beauty tip: You can use flaxseed oil combined with a drizzle of natural scent in the bath. It's not only relaxing but effective as a moisturizer for the skin.

1 TABLESPOON WHOLE FLAXSEEDS: 55 calories
1 TABLESPOON FLAXSEED OIL: 120 calories

HEMP SEEDS: They won't make you high, but these seeds (similar in taste to pine nuts) contain all nine of the essential amino acids. That makes them a perfect protein with nutritional properties very similar to egg whites. Hemp seeds are also a major source of essential fatty acids. But that's not all: Hemp seeds offer 45 percent of our daily magnesium requirement. Magnesium keeps our bones strong and can lower blood pressure and thanks to its calming effects can also help us sleep through the night. According to a 2010 study, a diet rich in magnesium can slash diabetes risk by almost half, possibly because it increases insulin sensitivity.

2 TABLESPOONS HEMP SEEDS: 90 calories

SUNFLOWER SEEDS: These crunchy and superyummy seeds are not only readily available, they're versatile and their health benefits are impressive. Sunflower seeds can help in preventing cancer by controlling cell damage. Their secret weapon? Selenium. They also contain plenty of bone–healthy minerals, including a combination of magnesium and copper. For glowing skin, sunflower seeds come to the rescue with an abundance of vitamin E, which helps to combat harmful UV rays. And sunflowers not only help prevent "bad" cholesterol from blocking our heart's arteries, they improve brain function thanks to their high levels of tryptophan, which increases the brain's production of stress–reducing serotonin.

¼ CUP SUNFLOWER SEEDS: 180 calories

WHEAT GERM: Are you wondering why wheat germ is included in the seed section? Well, wheat germ is actually the part of a grain that will develop into a seed. For refined grains like white bread and most processed snack foods, the germ is removed so you only get the starchy "endosperm," and that's what makes most commercially produced wheat a nutritional bummer. It's the "germ" that contains a high concentration of nutrients (a whopping 23), including niacin, thiamin, riboflavin, folate, vitamin E, magnesium, phosphorus, potassium, iron, and zinc. Wheat germ also provides dietary fiber and healthy fats to help balance blood sugar levels, control cholesterol levels, and promote intestinal health. Plus it supplies about 12 percent of your daily value of folate, the B vitamin believed to protect against colon cancer, stroke, cardiovascular disease, and dementia.

1 TABLESPOON WHEAT GERM: 120 calories

Fruits

Did you know?
At least 3,000 fruits are found in the rainforests; of these, only 200 are now in use in the Western World. In contrast, the indigenous people of the rainforest use over 2,000 fruit varieties.

APPLES: Who knows if an apple a day *really* keeps the doctor away, but one thing is for sure: One study found that folks who substituted all sugary sweets in their diet with apples lost an average of 15 pounds in 12 weeks. What's more, the fiber and pectin in this fruit protect our bodies against pollution and can relieve indigestion, gout, rheumatism, arthritis, and hangovers. Scientists from the American Association for Cancer Research agree that the consumption of flavonol-rich apples could also help reduce your risk of developing pancreatic cancer by up to 23 percent, and researchers at Cornell University identified several compounds in apple peel that have potent antigrowth activities against cancer cells in the liver, colon, and breast. In addition, a recent study performed on mice shows that drinking apple juice could keep Alzheimer's away by fighting the effects of aging on the brain. Mice in the study that were fed an apple-enhanced diet showed higher levels of the neurotransmitter acetylcholine and did better in maze tests than those on a regular diet.

1 MEDIUM APPLE WITH SKIN: 72 calories

AVOCADOS: Don't worry about the fat content in an avocado; most of its fat is the heart-healthy monounsaturated type. Avocados are an excellent source of vitamin E, which helps keep the heart in tip top shape by preventing the oxidation of LDL ("bad") cholesterol. One small avocado also provides over half the RDA of vitamin B6, which is essential for a healthy nervous system. Avocados contain the carotenoid lutein an antioxidant that specializes in protecting the eyes from oxidative stress damage leading to poor vision, cataracts, and macular degeneration. They also possess a high content of potassium along with omega-3 and oleic acid; all are beneficial toward reducing blood pressure. If you're worried about blood sugar levels, look to the avocado. Its monounsaturated fats can prevent or reverse insulin resistance, a source of type-2 diabetes. That's because the high soluble fiber of avocado helps prevent blood sugar spikes.

1 CUP SLICED AVOCADO: 234 calories

BLACK CURRANTS: A 1-cup serving of dried black currants contains 9.8 grams of dietary fiber. This amount supplies approximately 39 percent of the recommended daily allowance of fiber. These tiny berries also offer three times as much vitamin C as oranges do. Plus, they're rich in antioxidants known as bioflavonoids, which help to boost the immune system. Even better, they're a low-fat, cholesterol-free, and high-protein taste treat. Currants rank high as an excellent source of copper, manganese, and potassium. Research shows that a diet that regularly incorporates plenty of potassium-rich foods like dried currants may decrease the risk of osteoporosis, kidney disease, and stroke.

1 CUP BLACK CURRANTS: 71 calories

BLUEBERRIES: When it comes to neutralizing free radicals and protecting the body from premature aging, heart disease, cancer, and degenerative diseases, blueberries are on the top of the list. Blueberries have also been found to contain a chemical that may be as good at lowering cholesterol as some popular prescription drugs. As you probably know by now (but it's worth repeating), cholesterol is that fatty substance in the blood that can build up on the walls of the arteries and cause heart disease and stroke. These popular berries also offer heaps of the trace mineral manganese, which fights free radicals. According to the University of Maryland Medical Center, manganese may decrease premenstrual syndrome symptoms, improve bone health, reduce arthritis pain, and offer protection from low-density lipoprotein cholesterol in diabetics.

1 CUP BLUEBERRIES: 83 calories

COCONUT: Want to support your immune system? Eat coconut. It's antiviral, antifungal, antibacterial, and antiparasitic, meaning the nutrients in coconuts can kill harmful bacteria, viruses, fungi, and parasites. Because of that, if you consume coconut in any of its various forms (whether it's raw coconut,

coconut oil, coconut milk, coconut butter, etc.), it can help treat some of the world's most resilient illnesses such as influenza, giardia, lice, throat infections, urinary tract infections, tapeworms, herpes, gonorrhea, bronchitis, and numerous other ailments caused by microbials. Whether you're eating the meat, drinking the juice, or consuming it as oil, coconuts are also a delicious and nutritious source of fiber, vitamins, minerals, and amino acids. They have tons of calcium, potassium, and magnesium, as well as plenty of electrolytes. In fact, coconut water is known to have the same electrolyte levels as human plasma.

1 CUP SHREDDED COCONUT: 238 calories
1 (8-OUNCE) GLASS COCONUT MILK: 34 calories

GOJI BERRIES: New to the health-conscious Western consumer, these red-orange berries (also known as wolfberries) are native to China and Tibet and have been used medically for thousands of years in Asian countries. Although there are lots of goji berry drinks available, if you want the max in nutritional benefits, it's best to eat them in their most natural, unprocessed form. This superfood offers high levels of antioxidants, which are extremely effective in fighting cancer. Another benefit of antioxidants is that they can protect the heart from disease because they help in lowering cholesterol. Plus, goji berries contain fiber, and we all know how great that is. But maybe best of all, goji berries have been linked with wrinkle reduction and an overall slowing down of the aging process. In addition, this fruit contains vitamin A, zeaxanthin, and beta-carotene, all of which have been associated with healthier eyes.

½ CUP GOJI BERRIES: 177 calories

GRAPES: Grapes are fun to eat and easy to take along, and that's probably why they're among our most popular fruits. Good thing, because grapes are packed with lots of health-promoting phytonutrients such as polyphenolic antioxidants, vitamins, and minerals. Grapes also contain antioxidants in the form of flavonoids that work to increase the amount of good cholesterol in our system. Red grapes, in particular, contain resveratrol, which helps combat the aging process by limiting the natural cell damage that occurs to our bodies as we get older. What's more, if your doctor has prescribed a diuretic, you may be able to substitute a serving of grapes instead of the medication. That's because these little wonders have high levels of potassium and potassium salts, both of which act as natural diuretics.

1 CUP GRAPES: 62 calories

GRAPEFRUIT: So what if it's not the sweetest guy on the block? Sour grapefruit is worth its pucker. It contains plenty of minerals that help with detoxification in the liver. Grapefruit is high in vitamin C (which boosts the production of white blood cells) and increases the glutathione levels in red blood cells. If you dig into pink or red grapefruit, you'll get even more vitamin A, iron, and vitamin C than white grapefruit. Red grapefruit is also higher in antioxidants than white grapefruit. Full of fiber, no matter which color, it helps reduce LDL, or "bad," cholesterol.

Grapefruit Alert:
There are approximately 85 different drugs with which grapefruit can have a negative interaction. If you're on meds, get approval from your health care provider before including this fruit during your fast days.

1 AVERAGE PINK OR RED GRAPEFRUIT: 52 calories
1 AVERAGE WHITE GRAPEFRUIT: 39 calories

KIWI: Hairy and just a little strange looking, kiwi holds the title of "SUPER–C"! It has twice the vitamin C of an orange and as much potassium as a banana. That's pretty impressive, but its kiwi's lutein level that really packs a punch. Lutein is an antioxidant that appears to protect against macular degeneration, the leading cause of impaired vision in seniors. The hairy fruit is also rich in vitamins A and E, and it's full of phytonutrients, flavonoids, and carotenoids, which all provide antioxidant protection. Need fiber? Opt for a kiwi. It will give you more than if you chewed on four sticks of boring celery.

1 AVERAGE KIWI: 42 calories

ORANGES: Oranges are not only high in vitamin C, but they're also sources of key nutrients such as beta-carotene and folic acid. In fact, oranges contain more than 170 different phytochemicals and 60 flavonoids, many of which have disease-fighting properties. Oranges and other citrus fruits can play an important role in cancer prevention and seem to give the most powerful protection against mouth, throat, and stomach cancers. Research suggests that regularly eating citrus fruits could reduce the risk by 40 to 50 percent. Hint: Don't discard the peel; save it for uses such as zesting. Studies show that substances found in the peel of oranges and other citrus fruits can lower levels of harmful LDL cholesterol. The same substances are also found in the juice of the fruit, but in much smaller amounts.

1 AVERAGE ORANGE: 45 calories

WATERMELON: Know anyone who doesn't *love* luscious, thirst-quenching watermelon, especially on a hot summer day? It's sweet, juicy, refreshing, and best of all, very low in calories. That's because it's made up of 90 percent water, which means it's also a natural diuretic. Filled to the brim with vitamins, watermelon is an excellent source of the antistressor vitamin B6, as well as abundant in vitamin A. It's also rich in the carotenoid lycopene; studies point to lycopene's beneficial effect on prostate health. Watermelon also has immune-boosting antioxidant power because of its high level of glutathione, considered to be the body's most important antioxidant because it's found in every single one of our cells. Bonus: Watermelon seed kernels are also a good source of both potassium and magnesium.

1 SLICE WATERMELON: 85 calories

Vegetables

Question: What's the fastest vegetable?
Answer: A runner bean.

BEANS: As well as being an excellent source of fiber, beans can lower cholesterol and protect against osteoporosis, heart disease, diabetes, and cancers, including bowel, breast, and prostate. They're rich in protease inhibitors, compounds that may help slow the development of cancer cells. Beans also fight harmful free radicals because they're high in antioxidants. And here's surprising news: Studies show beans can prevent menstrual and menopausal symptoms. Soy beans are particularly beneficial for women with hormonal problems. And maybe best of all, even though they're a protein food, they won't bulk you up. In fact, beans provide little to no fat and are cholesterol-free. That's why they actually lower cholesterol and triglyceride levels instead of potentially causing them to increase as some animal proteins have been shown to do.

1 CUP BLACK BEANS: 218 calories
1 CUP PINTO BEANS: 206 calories
1 CUP RED KIDNEY BEANS: 218 calories
1 CUP SOY BEANS: 298 calories

BROCCOLI: A nutrition-packed veggie, broccoli goes the whole nine yards with vitamins, minerals, trace elements, fiber, calcium, and antioxidants. Looking and acting like the tree of life, broccoli's powerful anticarcinogenic properties stimulate the body to produce its own cancer-fighting substances. But broccoli doesn't stop there; it can also help prevent cataracts, heart disease, arthritis, ulcers, and viruses. The secret is to cook it lightly so that it doesn't lose its sulforaphane, a substance that causes the release of proteins that work to protect the body's cardiovascular system.

1 CUP CHOPPED BROCCOLI: 30 calories

CABBAGE: Korean, Chinese, and Swedish studies show that people eating lots of cabbage have lower rates of lung, colon, breast, and uterine cancers thanks to its cancer-protective glucosinolates and high levels of vitamins and minerals. Fiber-related components in cabbage also do an excellent job of binding together with bile acids in your digestive tract when they've been steamed. Cabbage is a good detoxifier, too. It purifies blood and removes toxins, primarily free radicals and uric acid. The presence of vitamin C and sulfur contribute to cabbage's detoxifying effects. It's rich in iodine and aids in proper functioning of the brain and the nervous system.

1 CUP CHOPPED RAW CABBAGE: 22 calories

CARROTS: What's up, Doc? Well, Bugs Bunny might not know that the versatile carrot could play a role in fighting wrinkles. According to the British Nutrition Foundation, vitamin A is essential to the normal function and structure of the skin, and carrots are a good source of beta-carotene, which the body converts into vitamin A. Beta-carotene has also been shown to protect against macular degeneration and cataracts. A study found that people who eat the most beta-carotene had a 40 percent lower risk of macular degeneration than those who consumed little. And studies have shown the falcarinol and falcarindiol in carrots reduce the risk of lung, breast, and colon cancers. The regular consumption of carrots also reduces cholesterol levels because the soluble fibers in the vegetable bind with bile acids.

1 MEDIUM RAW CARROT: 35 calories

CHICKPEAS (GARBANZO BEANS): As well as being a good source of low-fat protein, chickpeas are rich in soluble fiber. This helps to lower cholesterol and protect against diabetes and has been shown to help prevent heart disease. A major U.S. study followed 10,000 adults for 19 years and found those who ate the most fiber had a significantly lower risk of heart disease and stroke than those who ate very little. The heart-protective properties of chickpeas don't stop there. They also contain potassium, which can help lower blood pressure, and its folic acid reduces blood levels of homocysteine, thought to increase the risk of heart disease and stroke. The soluble fiber in chickpeas may also protect against certain cancers, particularly bowel cancer.

1 CUP CHICKPEAS: 269 calories

GARLIC: Where to begin? The prince of healers, garlic has proved itself to have antiviral, antifungal, and antibiotic properties in numerous studies. A study at the University of California found that garlic juice had a powerful effect against a wide range of antibiotic-resistant bacteria, including the hospital superbug MRSA. Garlic may also protect against heart disease. One large German study found that patients given garlic powder had a significant reduction in blood cholesterol levels, while other research suggests it may help lower blood pressure. Garlic is also known to help prevent blood clots. There's also mounting evidence that it's a potent anticancer agent since findings from China show that eating a lot of garlic lowers the risk of stomach cancer. Hint: When preparing garlic, chop or crush it to trigger the release of allicin, the substance responsible for some of garlic's health benefits. To allow for maximum allicin production, scientists recommend waiting 15 minutes between peeling, crushing, or chopping and cooking or eating. Did I mention it's really low in calories?

1 CLOVE RAW GARLIC: 4 calories

LEAFY GREENS: Spinach, kale, collards, Swiss chard, mustard greens – *whatever* – leafy green vegetables are powerful superfoods packed with vitamin C, beta-carotene, folic acid, and fiber, as well as being a good source of calcium, which protects bones against osteoporosis. Leafy vegetables, particularly spinach and kale, are also rich in lutein and zeaxanthin, two antioxidants called carotenoids. Research has shown a high intake of these reduces the risk of cataracts, and a U.S. National Eye Institute study found that eating a lot of food rich in carotenoids was linked with a reduced risk of age-related macular degeneration. Green leafy veggies, especially kale, can also help protect against cancer, thanks to substances they contain called isothiocyanates, which have been shown to boost the body's ability to fight the disease. Green vegetables also have plenty of calcium. Although there are many factors that influence whether you'll develop osteoporosis, such as exercise and hormone levels, sufficient calcium in the diet is a crucial element.

1 CUP SPINACH: 7 calories

1 CUP KALE: 33 calories

1 CUP SWISS CHARD: 7 calories

1 CUP MUSTARD GREENS: 21 calories

RADISHES: Rich in glucosinolates, radishes help ward off cancer while maintaining a healthy liver and gall bladder. They're also full of vitamin C, folic acid, potassium, and selenium. A radish's pungent flavor and natural spice can help eliminate excess mucus in the body, and it's especially helpful when fighting a cold. What's more, radishes cannot only help clear the sinuses and soothe sore throats, but they're a natural cleansing agent for the digestive system, helping to break down and eliminate stagnant food and toxins that built up over time.

1 SERVING RADISHES (ABOUT 7): 15 calories

SHIITAKE MUSHROOMS: If you're a stickler for the definition of "vegetable," strictly speaking, shiitakes don't belong in this category because mushrooms are a fungus. But for the sake of simplicity, let's include this health-packed, low-calorie mushroom here. Used medicinally by the Chinese for more than 6,000 years, they not only contain phytochemicals, which are believed to help strengthen the immune system by stimulating white blood cell production, but other studies show they can help lower high blood cholesterol levels. Plus, they contain lots of B vitamins and iron. Did I say they're yummy? That too.

1 WHOLE SHIITAKE MUSHROOM: 6 calories

SWEET POTATOES: Just one of these gems provides over 100 percent of the recommended daily amount (RDA) of vitamin E–that's 50 times more than white potatoes. They also provide excellent amounts of beta–carotene (which the body converts to vitamin A) and vitamin C. While most of us know that vitamin C is important to help ward off cold and flu viruses, few people are aware that it's crucial in bone and tooth formation, for keeping digestion optimum, and in blood cell formation. It also helps accelerate wound healing, produces collagen, which helps maintain skin's youthful elasticity, and is essential to helping us cope with stress. It even appears to help protect our body against toxins that may be linked to cancer. Sweet potatoes also offer the important minerals copper, iron, potassium, and magnesium.

1 MEDIUM SWEET POTATO: 114 calories

FYI:
Magnesium is necessary for healthy artery, blood, bone, heart, muscle, and nerve function, yet experts estimate that approximately 80 percent of our population may be deficient in this important mineral.

TOMATOES: Scientifically speaking, a tomato is a fruit, but let's call it a vegetable since it's so often used in savory rather than sweet dishes, not to mention in salads and sliced for sandwiches. Tomatoes are the rock stars of superfoods. They're the richest source of the supernutrient lycopene, which is known to protect against breast and prostate cancers and is essential for avoiding vision loss in old age. American researchers tracked nearly 40,000 middle-aged and older women over five years and found that as lycopene levels in their blood went up, their risk of heart disease and stroke dropped. Low lycopene levels have been linked with several cancers, including bowel and prostate. Scottish researchers have also found that the yellow jelly around tomato seeds helps make blood less prone to clotting. Tomatoes contain other protective phytochemicals, and scientists think it's the combination of these that provides the best protection for overall health.

1 AVERAGE TOMATO: 116 calories

WATERCRESS: Are you old enough to remember those snooty watercress sandwiches? Well, you don't have to be an heiress to enjoy one. Widely regarded as one of the oldest superfoods, watercress is rich in folate, iron, calcium, vitamins A, C, and E, lutein, and quercetin. Highly nutritious, watercress has a peppery, slightly hot flavor that is somewhat reduced when it's cooked. Gram for gram, watercress contains 12 times more vitamin C than lettuce and more iron than spinach. It's also rich in several of the B vitamins, beta-carotene, magnesium, and potassium. Watercress contains a host of phytochemcials, many of which have been shown to have powerful anticancer properties. Studies have also shown that watercress may help to prevent colorectal cancer.

1 CUP CHOPPED WATERCRESS: 4 calories

Which Superfoods Do You Need Most?

Sure we all need to eat to live, but our bodies and temperaments are different. Some of us are high-strung, get stressed out, go on hyper-drive, love a challenge, dig competitive exercising, and are practical and hands-on, while others get fatigued easily, take it slow, retreat rather than confront difficulties, would rather walk than run, are dreamy and imaginative, and enjoy nothing more than curling up on the couch with a good book. These are personality traits, but they give clues to the kind of superfoods our bodies are craving. Experts say if you don't have the right eating plan in place, you'll be three times as likely to go off your diet. This quiz identifies the superfoods that match your personality and lifestyle. Use it to get the most out of your Two-Day Superfood Cleanse.

Quiz
Discover *Your* Top Superfoods

1. While on the job I'm more apt to:
   a. Welcome interruptions.
   b. Allow for interruptions, but I don't really enjoy them.
   c. Let others know in advance I prefer not to be interrupted.

2. My idea of comfort dining is:
   a. Anything delivered.
   b. Something sweet and gooey.
   c. A three-course meal served in a restaurant.

3. When I feel the sniffles coming on, I'm most likely to:
   a. Ignore it and carry on.
   b. Take an over-the-counter remedy.
   c. Cuddle up on the couch, keeping tissues and hot tea within reach.

4. **If I'm channel surfing, I'll likely stop on a:**
   a. *Reality show or the news.*
   b. *Crime or medical drama.*
   c. *Classic movie or sitcom.*

5. **My dream vacation would be a:**
   a. *Whirlwind five-city tour of Europe.*
   b. *Cross-country trip in fully equipped RV.*
   c. *Relaxing week at a slow-paced beach resort.*

6. **While driving along the highway, you'll find me putting my pedal to the metal in the:**
   a. *Fast lane.*
   b. *Middle lane.*
   c. *Slow lane.*

7. **During my lunch hour on my last hectic work day, I:**
   a. *Happily ate at my desk.*
   b. *Got out for a short breather.*
   c. *Took the full hour off — I needed a break.*

8. **Which meal would you prepare for guests?**
   a. *A risky dish I've never tried before but is guaranteed to make an impression.*
   b. *Something complicated that I've already mastered.*
   c. *A simple tried-and-true menu I'm sure everyone will enjoy.*

9. **I would prefer to celebrate my birthday with:**
   a. *A big bash that was a total surprise.*
   b. *A well-planned get-together shared with my loved ones.*
   c. *An intimate dinner with a person I adore.*

Mostly A's

You enjoy the blast of the last minute and the race to the finish line. And with a schedule as packed as yours, it may seem like good news that you're a master at rushing around, multitasking, and waiting until the last possible second to tackle big projects. But when you play beat the clock and don't budget your time, you're bound to feel stressed out, and stress causes magnesium loss. The following superfoods are rich in magnesium and geared for go-getter types like you:

- Wheat germ
- Buck wheat
- Garbanzo beans
- Spinach
- Almonds

Lifestyle changes:

- Set doable daily goals. The longer your list, the less you're likely to accomplish and the more stressed out you'll feel.

- Learn to take a breather and relax. Hyper-schedulers like you often view downtime as wasted time. It's not. Ask yourself: "What's really important in my life?" This simple question can help you set important priorities.

- Shut down distractions and limit multitasking. Studies show when you don't give full attention to a primary task you'll make 30 percent more mistakes and can spend up to 20 percent more time correcting them.

- Schedule time for pleasure. Stress junkies have a hard time sitting still, so recharge by making fun-packed dates with friends and family.

Mostly B's

You've learned the secret to keeping stress in balance by looking at the big picture and not allowing yourself to get caught up in nit-picking details. It's all about setting priorities, feeling guilt-free when you do take time for yourself, and making sure your expectations aren't on overdrive. For the most part, you're already on the right track, but be honest: Don't you feel like you have to be the one in control? Focusing on these superfoods that contain hefty levels of B and E vitamins will help bolster your balance.

- Broccoli
- Sweet potatoes
- Avocados
- Pine nuts

Lifestyle changes:

- Delegate. Allow others who have expertise to carry some of the load. If it makes you uncomfortable to let someone else share responsibility, it's okay to check in once in a while.

- Open your palms. Surprisingly, a study shows this simple gesture of letting go actually helps release the impulse to take over situations.

- Have a plan B. Psychologists say being prepared for change is the best way to prevent stress around it. When writing out your to-do list, pencil in alternatives.

Mostly C's

Since you easily opt for relaxation before accomplishment, chores and responsibilities can mount up until you finally can't help but feel overwhelmed. It can be a messy house, a stack of unpaid bills, or clutter on your desk. In the end, you feel overwhelmed and that's when your immune system gets walloped. What you need in terms of a superfood diet is to focus on those edibles that boost your immune system so you won't fall prey to colds, the flu, or that rundown feeling. Focus on these immune-boosting superfoods:

- Garlic
- Blueberries, black currants, kiwis, oranges
- Flax, hemp, and chia seeds
- Carrots

Lifestyle changes:

- Create a special place for everything and put things away before they get out of hand.

- Make a list of actions or goals you need to reach and then give yourself a deadline to achieve them. When you take actions step by step, you'll be less likely to feel overwhelmed.

- Say "yes" instead of "no." Your first reaction may be to turn down a challenge, but think it over again. Exploring different options can actually expand your ability to cope.

- Try tai chi, yoga, or meditation. You have the perfect personality for these proven stress–relieving practices. Plus, each of them can help you learn to stay focused as well as calm.

2

Losing It

Diets, like clothes, should be tailored to you.
                                    ~Joan Rivers

It probably surprises no one that we're a nation of obsessed dieters. We'll do just about anything–from sucking up grapefruit juice or just drinking cabbage soup to chewing every bite 32 times or consuming a diet of cavemen food–in order to lose those extra pounds. And who can blame us? We want to drop that belly-rolling, arm-sagging jiggle weight. In the process we're willing to try, try, try … and try again. According to NPD, a market research company that collected its National Eating Trends (NET) data through telephone surveys of approximately 5,000 Americans in 2,000 households, 23 percent of women say they've been on a diet at some point during the year. The report also suggests we're giving up on our diets much quicker than ever before, in fact, in a heartbeat.

All this crazy yo-yo dieting can put our health into a tailspin. Some studies suggest that weight cycling can increase the risk for certain physical problems. These include high blood pressure, high cholesterol, and gallbladder disease. If you're not obese and don't have weight–related health problems, crazy dieting can still have a negative psychological effect if you let yourself become discouraged or depressed when the weight returns. Most experts recommend maintaining a stable weight to avoid any potential risks associated with this kind of yo–yo approach.

What's the message? Want to lose weight (and who doesn't)? Better do it in a hurry and do it right the first time.

The good news is that there are awesome techniques to get you there quicker than you can say lickety–split or lick your lips. The downside? Not every method is both good for your body *and* for your soul. So, let's look at the absolute best approach to dieting and weigh in on its pros and cons.

Fading In and Out: The Best Diet

My pick for the best way to shed pounds is with the wildly successful "Fast Diet," but be prepared for some tweaking. The Fast Diet, also known as the 5:2 Diet, was devised by a duo of British broadcasting journalists, Michael Mosley and Mimi Spencer. What makes their approach so appealing and ultimately successful is that it allows participants to eat whatever they desire for five days of the week. In case you're thinking, "Oh yeah, what about a burger and fries?" The answer is *Yes!* "Pizza topped with everything?" *Yes!* "Fried whole belly clams?" *Yes!* "Ice cream sundae?" *Yes! Yes! Yes!* Okay, so you get the idea. You can eat ANYTHING. Go whole hog.

Of course, there's a hitch and this is it: During two nonconsecutive days of the week, dieters can only consume 600 calories (about a quarter of a normal healthy adult's intake). Moseley has explained that the diet is based on work by British and U.S. scientists who found intermittent fasting helped people lose more fat, increase insulin sensitivity, and cut cholesterol. As an experiment, Moseley tried this eating regimen himself for a BBC television science program called "Eat, Fast, Live Longer." Guess what? Over a three month period he lost a whopping 18 pounds.

The creators of the diet insist that one of the biggest reasons their 5:2 approach is so successful is that it leads to a steady drop in weight with an average weekly loss of one pound for women and a bit more for guys. (Any diet promoting more than a one- or two-pound weight loss a week means most of it is going to be fluid. It's almost impossible to lose more weight steadily unless you weigh, like, 500 pounds.) Plus, on this plan you only have to be on a diet two days a week. You choose the days so it's flexible and easy because–and this is worth repeating–you can eat *anything* and *any amount* when you're not fasting.

Plus, the British Dietetic Association (BDA) reviewed a 2011 study by researchers at the UK's University Hospital of South Manchester that suggested intermittent fasting could help lower the risk of certain obesity-related cancers such as breast cancer.

What could go wrong? Let's put down those knives and forks and take a hard look at a big part of the diet–those two days when you're keeping your calories below 600, engaging in a type of fast.

Traditional Fasting

Did you know?
Renowned Indian nationalist leader Mahatma Gandhi fasted a total of 17 times throughout his career.

By definition, fasting is the act of voluntary abstention or dramatic reduction of food, drink, or both for a period of time, usually a day or two. Humans have been using this practice of deprivation for millennia. In the earliest times, we had no choice. Sometimes there was food available, let's say if a hunter's arrow pierced a wandering yak, and other times, not so much. What's more, when you think about it, every animal fasts when they're stressed out or sick. It's just plain natural for *all* beings, whether human or animal, to seek rest and balance, as well as to conserve energy at critical times in their life.

The great early philosophers, including Hippocrates, Plato, Socrates, and Aristotle, promoted the benefits of fasting. Ancient religious and spiritual groups also used fasting as a part of ceremonies and rite, most often during spring and fall equinoxes. Today, every single major religion practices fasting for various spiritual benefit, including Christianity, Judaism, Gnosticism, Islam, Buddhism, Hinduism, as well as South and North American Indian traditions. Lots of these faiths prescribe regular fasting to prevent or break the habits of gluttony. Yogic practices, including that of fasting, date back thousands of years.

Fasting is indicated prior to surgery or other procedures that require general anesthetics. Certain medical tests, such as cholesterol and glucose measurements, as well as thyroid levels, may also require fasting for a full 12 hours to get accurate results.

Voluntarily withholding sustenance, a so-called hunger strike, is used fairly frequently to make a political statement or to bring about social justice. Perhaps the most famous faster was India's political and religious leader, Mahatma Gandhi, who engaged in several periods of fasting. There are other well-known political fasters, including Ireland's Bobby Sands, who was part of the 1981 British hunger strike, and Cesar Chavez, who went on a 25-day fast in 1968 to promote the principle of nonviolence. Presently, there are frequent protest fasts at Guantanamo Bay prison.

And, of course, fasting helps us lose weight. Scientifically it works like this: In order to lose weight you need to take in fewer and fewer calories. In other words, you need to create a caloric deficit. Fasting also helps increase fat oxidation while protecting lean mass. What does this mean? Well, besides losing weight we also want to lose fat—you know, that roll around your middle. Fasting increases those fat-burning hormones while decreasing hormones that inhibit fat burning. Another benefit: Studies show you're more likely to stick to a diet if it includes fasting as part of its plan. So, it sounds like a no-brainer. Right? Not so fast (ha ha). Abstaining from food can also be a bummer.

It's estimated that 14 percent of U.S. adults have reported using fasting as a means to control body weight.

What's the Problem with Straight-Forward, Conventional Fasting?

KICKS YOU INTO SURVIVAL MODE: When you're fasting and your body isn't getting the proper nutrients, it drives itself into self-preservation mode to counter starvation. It can begin to not only slow down your metabolism but also bump up the production of the stress hormone cortisol, which is manufactured by your adrenal glands. A high amount of cortisol surging through your body can make you feel physically, mentally, and/or emotionally stressed out while the flight-or-fight mechanism is switched on. These days, no one needs to feel even more fried.

DAMAGES MUSCLES: When your body isn't taking in enough nutrition, it will try to release certain amino acids from your muscles and then convert them into sugar. The sugar not only surges to your brain but also to your kidneys and red blood cells. By releasing amino acids, your muscle tissue can begin to break down, which ultimately can slow weight loss. How come? Because you need muscles to burn that excess fat.

GETS YOU SICK: Conventional fasting can deplete your supply of essential nutrients such as proteins, vitamins, minerals, and electrolytes. This can lead to various health issues, including fatigue, headache, dizziness, constipation, hypoglycemia, anemia, muscle weakness, gallstones, and mental confusion. This is why if you're already suffering with *any* kind of health problem, it's a good idea for you to kiss the idea of fasting good-bye. At the very least, speak with your doctor about it.

GIVES FUEL TO OBSESSION: Fasting can cause people to think too much about food, and ironically overeat on the days when they're allowed to eat freely. If people eat lots of cake and cookies on their "normal eating" days and don't think about their overall diet, it can potentially lead to nutrient deficiencies and poor eating habits. This can lead to eating disorders; susceptible folks might develop eating disorders while on the diet, and engage in starvation, binging, or both.

FASTING MAY CREATE AN ABNORMAL PHYSIOLOGICAL STATE: Those who adopt fasting as a means of weight loss and not healthy cleansing can ultimately end up developing gastrointestinal problems. That's because your body has peak times for secretion of digestive enzymes (at breakfast, lunch, and dinner). In the absence of food, these enzymes keep circulating within and damage the lining of the digestive tract. This can lead to acid reflux, gastritis problems, and even ulcers.

COMPROMISES IMMUNITY: When you don't eat, your intestinal tract (responsible for over 70 percent of your antibodies) stops working for your immune system. In the absence of antibodies, bacteria, toxins, and viruses can suddenly have an easier time staying alive inside your gut. When the raw material necessary for an intestinal tract (sufficient vitamins and minerals) is missing, your immunity is shot.

Well, you might ask, should fasting be taken off the table? Answer: Serve the Superfood Cleanse instead!

What Is the Superfood Cleanse?

A modified fast that cleanses the body of accumulated toxins and enriches it through a diet of low-calorie, highly nutritious superfoods is the way to go. This kind of detox cleansing will get the same positive calorie-reducing effects as a 5:2-type diet, but rather than putting your health at risk, it promotes a whopping heart-healthy, beauty-enhancing, energy-enlivening boost. You'll look younger, feel better, have more get up and go, maintain your muscles, and at the same time, avoid the negative side effects of conventional fasting. You'll also lose weight at the same clip as a conventional fast, but you'll stay healthier because you're using, not abusing, your body by making nutritional, low-calorie choices that fully support your physical, mental, and emotional well-being during your fasting days.

Superfoods build bones, prevent chronic diseases, improve your eyesight, and even keep your mind sharp. There's also evidence to suggest that these kinds of foods can help you stay slimmer longer because your body isn't craving nutrition and beckoning you to binge.

High-quality food is better for your health.

~ Michael Pollan

Why Cleanse? It's a Dirty World: Go Clean

Exposure to toxins is part of our everyday lives. We can thank modern chemistry for introducing lots of harmful toxins into our environment. These top ten everyday toxins are just a drop in the filthy bucket. Even though this is a grim report, keep in mind that the Two-Day Superfood Cleanse is an excellent way to counteract damage. The secret is to take the opportunity to choose these foods during your low-calorie fast and purge icky toxins from your body.

PRESCRIPTION DRUGS: Sadly, whatever goes down our drains ends up in the public water supply. The United States Environmental Protection Agency (EPA) has found trace amounts of pharmaceuticals, cosmetics, and even illegal drugs in municipal water supplies. For example, studies have shown that even tiny amounts of estrogen released via discarded birth control pills have affected male fish.

VOCS (VOLATILE ORGANIC COMPOUNDS): These are found in plenty of household products and include acetone, formaldehyde, and turpentine. VOC exposure can cause respiratory irritation and memory impairment, as well as allergic and immune reactions. VOCs are also suspected cancer-causing agents in humans. Household VOCs are found in cleaning fluids, carpets, and paints. VOCs are by-products of protective coatings and may contribute to what has been referred to as Sick Building Syndrome.

PERCHLORATE: This substance is used in a wide range of products from thyroid medications to rocket fuel. Its chief hazard in the human body is its ability to block iodine uptake, which has been linked to thyroid ailments and can be especially harmful to the unborn fetus. Perchlorate has been found in water sources near military bases and chemical plants. Plus, any perchlorates wind up in our environment from their use in fertilizers and explosives, including fireworks. Perchlorates from construction demolition and fertilizers leech into the soil from runoff, and are then incorporated into plants and later concentrated in grazing animals.

ASBESTOS: You've heard about this, but maybe you think it's already been eliminated. Think again. Asbestos is a naturally occurring fibrous silicate material. Asbestos was used for years because of its heat-resistant and insulation properties before its more insidious nature became known. Asbestos inhalation causes malignant lung cancer in the form of mesothelioma. It can still be found in drywall, pipe fittings, automotive brake and clutch parts, and even toys and fireplace logs, but it is most commonly found in housing and electrical insulation.

MOLDS: Molds are fungi that are common in warm, humid areas. In any home, the question is not if there is mold, but how much there is. Most mold and yeast spores are benign; large amounts can lead to respiratory concerns and reactions, especially among individuals with pre-existing immunodeficiency disorders. Also, mold may refer to anything including common molds and yeasts that are used in the production of medicine and fermentation of alcohol.

PHTHALATES: This compound is used anywhere flexibility and durability is desired. Some studies suggest that phthalates may be linked to endocrine disruption as well as increased birth defects in newborn males. Phthalate exposure is also suspected in elevated breast cancer rates. In the home, phthalates are present in shower curtains, toys, upholstery, and even the dissolvable coatings of medicines; in fact, anywhere soft, flexible rubber parts or coatings are used you'll find phthalates. Phthalates are also found in certain lotions, cosmetics, and shampoos.

PESTICIDES: Yes, DDT was banned in 1972 after the publication of *Silent Spring* by Rachael Carson, but it still shows up in the blood tests of many Americans decades later and can lead to impaired neurological development, diabetes, and breast cancer. DDT was used extensively to eliminate malaria–carrying mosquitoes up until the 1970s. Other pesticides are still used in agriculture and by pest treatment and lawn care services.

PCBS: Widely used in the U.S. as a coolant fluid for industrial electric equipment, polychlorinated biphenyls are persistent organic pollutants that can cause nervous and endocrine problems in the human body. PCBs have been linked to deadly forms of liver and brain cancer.

RADIOACTIVITY: Natural deposits of radon and uranium can be found in every U.S. state, and radon may even be present in the granite countertop in your kitchen. The EPA estimates that around 1 in 15 homes nationwide has elevated radon levels, and the agency cites radon with causing more than 20,000 cancer deaths per year. In addition to what leeches out naturally through the soil, a few atoms of non–naturally occurring plutonium are now present in each of our bodies, the result of mid–twentieth century nuclear testing.

HEAVY METALS: Element 48, or cadmium, is used in what we use plenty of: electronics. What makes this particular element so toxic is that it mimics one of our body's key nutrients, zinc, and thus our body unwittingly incorporates it into organs where it can wreak havoc. Other toxic elements include mercury, arsenic, lead, and even some forms of aluminum and nickel. Mercury is most often ingested by eating fish, particularly king mackerel, lake trout, and swordfish, which accumulate the element. Many older homes still contain lead–based paints. Other common sources of heavy metals include mining and smelting operations.

Superfoods have the power to remove metabolic waste, harmful chemicals, and other toxins from blood, organs, tissue, and fat cells.

How Does a Superfood Cleanse Work?

After a couple of days of *eating anything you want*, your body is probably ready to reduce your intake. According to the Fast Diet rules you can choose any two non-consecutive days to fast and keep your intake down to 600 calories. For example, you could choose to eat a couple of doughnuts, a container of yogurt and granola, a burger on a bun, a couple of slices of pizza, a small bag of chips and a hot dog, or a heaping portion of superfudge ice cream. You'll be meeting the 5:2 requirements, but you won't be doing your body any favors.

Instead, if on your calorie-limited days you opt for superfoods that contain organic and natural proteins, vitamins, minerals, bioflavonoids, and other naturally occurring essential cofactors that regenerate red blood cells and supply fresh oxygen to your body, you'll gain a powerful blast of immunity and energy. You'll not only continue to lose weight but your hair will shine, your face will glow, and you'll be bounding through the day, a vision of vitality.

But like every aspect of our lives, not all of us will approach wellness in the same way. Before moving on to the nitty-gritty of the Two-Day Superfood Cleanse, take this quick quiz to discover tips tailor-made for you.

Quiz
Discover the Personality Secrets in Your Favorite Foods

There's real truth to the old adage "you are what you eat"; our food choices hold clues to our core personalities. Take this quiz to find out what's *really* hiding in your food choices.

1. **When you order dessert at a restaurant it's usually:**
    a. *Really going to satisfy your sweet tooth — no holds barred!*
    b. *Yummy but not too high in calories; maybe pie.*
    c. *Nothing. You prefer to have dessert at home.*

2. **When you're feeling stressed, you would rather snack on:**
    a. *Chocolates or gummy bears.*
    b. *A bowl of ice cream.*
    c. *Nuts or fruit.*

3. **The last time you ate at a buffet, you:**
    a. *Tasted everything tempting, and maybe went back again.*
    b. *Chose a plate of your favorites.*
    c. *Stuck to veggies and dip.*

4. **Ideally, your favorite place to eat is:**
    a. *Anywhere different. You're up for trying out new restaurants.*
    b. *The family standby where you know you get the dish you like best!*
    c. *Your own kitchen — as long as someone else cleans up.*

5. **Driving home from a stressful chore, you would be most likely to snack on:**
    a. *Cookies or chips you keep in the car.*
    b. *An energy bar.*
    c. *Water or nothing.*

6. **The breakfast would you opt for is:**
    a. *Fruit tart or croissant.*
    b. *Bran muffin or cereal.*
    c. *Oatmeal with blueberries.*

7. **When you're thirsty, your choice of beverage is usually:**
    a. *Soda.*
    b. *Fruit juice or an energy drink.*
    c. *Water.*

8. The word that most closely fits your eating style is:
   a. Random.
   b. Predictable.
   c. Picky.

9. You would rather do without:
   a. Protein.
   b. Sugar.
   c. Salt.

10. What would you prefer to put on your pasta?
   a. An exotic spicy tomato sauce.
   b. Meat balls and lots of cheese.
   c. Creamy primavera.

Mostly A's: You're an Impatient Go-Getter

Outgoing and full of pep, you energize everyone around you. Your bubbly personality also inspires others to lighten up and seize the day with joy. Enthusiastic, energetic, and always up for something new and different, you tend to choose foods that are usually sweet and fast. Impulsive and full of spontaneity, you hate wasting time or worrying about what you're going to eat. That's why you'll opt for a quick fix to keep you going–usually a sweet. Your eating style means the Two-Day Superfood Cleanse may present special challenges. Try these tips:

- Keep a list of superfoods in your purse or pocket.

- Stock your cupboards and refrigerator for quick go-to superfoods.

- Make meditation a part of your day, even if it's just ten minutes. It will help you slow down and be more mindful.

Mostly B's: You're a Solid Realist

You always *try* to stay on schedule, meet your goals, and do what's best for you and your health – yet still have fun! Which means you won't make yourself crazy sticking to hard and fast rules. Your flexibility and willingness to compromise means you choose from a wide variety of foods, but your favorites are often tried-and-true comfort dishes like ice cream and mac and cheese. Studies show people who keep one eye on nutrition but don't feel guilty when they indulge are more likely to maintain a healthy weight—and be happier. FYI: Staying realistic about goals also means friends come to you for advice because they know they can depend on you to be smart and practical. You can use these techniques to help tame your natural tendency toward comfort foods:

- Drink plenty of water: Since cleansing is all about getting rid of toxins, you can help it along by flushing them out. Calorie intake: Zero.

- Let go of dairy: This food group is not cleanse-worthy. Surprisingly, even yogurt on a low-calorie day isn't a healthy choice. Why? Dairy products encourage toxin-holding mucous to form in your stomach, nose, and throughout your body.

- Exercise: You may not feel like being on the move on those low-calorie days, but opting for exercise will help you release acids and toxins from every pore on your skin.

Mostly C's: You're a Deep Thinker

You don't rely on anyone's judgment other than your own—and there's good reason for your self-confidence. You're a careful thinker, someone who weighs the pros and cons, takes her time, and looks at all sides of the equation. That's why you're keenly aware of nutritional facts and choose a diet based on what's healthiest. Plus, since it's your nature to delve deeply into matters, you prefer to plan and make your own meals; that way you know what's in the food you're eating. These tips can help you make the most of your natural tendency toward superfoods.

- Use herbs to give your body a boost: Certain herbs can up the ante of a Superfood Cleanse. For example, milk thistle is a proven liver-regenerator and detoxifier, while dandelion is a well-established kidney-restoring herb, and flaxseeds help eliminate toxic material from the intestines.

- Eliminate added sugar, alcohol, caffeine, wheat/gluten, eggs, animal protein, corn, and soy: These substances are allergens and need to be eliminated while you are doing a cleanse. Remind yourself to keep your metabolic process as clean and simple as possible.

- Drink to your health: Consider trading in a portion of your 600-calorie limit on a detoxifying smoothie. It's a great way to bump up your metabolism and boost your digestive system.

The ABC's of Cleansing

I really like to sometimes go into food detox and eat very simply.

~ Padma Lakshmi

Cleansing is exactly what it sounds like–a process that cleans your body so that it will sparkle inside and out. It works to eliminate all those accumulated toxins discussed in earlier chapters: the build-up from industrial chemicals, pesticides, additives in foods, secondary smoke, heavy metals, and other icky pollutants. And when the body is cleansed, so is the mind. While participating in your cleanse your emotions will settle down and you'll probably find yourself a lot more relaxed. During these days you'll also be more in control and much less likely to blow your cork. A cleanse brings you back to the center of your being, your truest calm-as-a-lake essence.

It may sound like a big deal–and it *is*–but on the other hand, it's easy-breezy because it's the natural order of things. Most of the cleansing takes place through your body's organs that are naturally devoted to detoxing, which includes your kidneys, skin, liver, lungs (through breath), and colon. And like most things in life, the more you do it, the easier it becomes. So, the more frequently you engage in detoxification, the more powerful the results. For example, once heavy metals are detoxed, other parasitic, yeast, and organic detoxing proceeds at a quicker and deeper rate.

How Do I Know if I Need to Cleanse?

These are common signs:

- Headaches
- Unexplained back pain
- Fuzzy brain
- Brittle and cracked nails
- Dry and lifeless hair
- Frequent allergies
- Hyper stress
- Moodiness or depression
- Digestive irregularity
- Insomnia
- Exposure to toxic solvents, pesticides, diuretics, and certain drugs, etc.

Basic Benefits of Superfood Cleansing

You'll experience:

- Higher energy levels
- Fewer food cravings

- Weight loss
- Improved mood
- Increased immune functions
- Sharper mind
- Shiny hair and glowing skin
- Overall relaxation

The Superfood Advantage

When superfoods are the mainstay of your cleanse, you up the health ante by boosting your immune system, balancing your hormones, and enhancing the benefits of detoxification not only in your liver, colon, and kidneys, but through blood purification as well. You'll also discover that any dependency you might have on substances such as sugar, caffeine, nicotine, or alcohol, is reduced. Superfoods subtly support your body and mind to move in the direction of pure wellness. They give your body *exactly* what it needs to go through the cleansing process with ease.

Calories Clarified

Most of us get a little crazy around calories, especially when we have to keep them extremely low during a diet. In the case of the 5:2 diet, we're talking about 600 calories or fewer on each of the two days, which is pretty minimal. So, let's keep the low-calorie business simple. Here's the scoop on calories 101:

Calories are just like any measuring tool. Think finding inches on a ruler. They measure the energy of every food or drink on the planet. Since calories are the fuel that keeps our bodies and minds working, of course we need to have them. They supply our body with energy in a similar way that gasoline keeps a car running.

The bummer is that foods and beverages vary in how many calories *and* nutrients they contain. When choosing what to eat and drink, it's important to get the right mix. In other words, you need enough nutrients but not too many calories. That's another way superfoods hit the exact spot. The benefit of choosing superfood fruits, vegetables, seeds, nuts, and grains is that you will definitely get more of a nutritious bang for your caloric buck.

A FACT OF LIFE

Any calories you consume above your suggested daily calorie intake will cause you to gain weight, while consuming fewer calories than your suggested daily calorie intake will cause you to lose weight. A pound is measured by 3,500 calories. So if you consume 3,500 more calories than you burn during a day, you'll gain a pound; if you burn 3,500 more calories than you consume during a day, you'll lose a pound.

Counting Calories

Of course you can find out the calories in foods by looking at the calorie label or the nutrition facts panel on packages, but most likely those are on processed food labels and won't be part of your Superfood Cleanse. There are also plenty of websites that tell you the calories of nearly every food on the planet. If you're a paper fancier, you can carry a pocket-sized book with calorie counts. Just make sure that after you check the calories for a serving size you only eat that much. So, get out those measuring spoons and cups to keep serving sizes exact!

To take the guesswork out of *your* Superfood Cleanse, calories are listed below the description of each food, and then again in the recipe section. Since practice makes perfect, there's a good chance that after a few weeks, you'll be a pro at knowing how many calories you're ingesting.

Remember: On your Superfood Cleanse the daily limit is 600 calories!

Hint:
Drink plenty of water. Water is essential for the health of your body's organs. Best of all, water contains absolutely no calories.

The Importance of Portions

CALORIES: One of the biggest reasons we need to watch portion size is to control our calorie intake. Ten almonds are good for your health, but a bowlful is a heap of bad. Even if you think you can skip a meal and then hunker down for the other two, research shows that people who eat only two to three large meals a day are more apt to become chunky than folks who eat more frequent, smaller meals.

BLOOD SUGAR LEVELS: If you eat smaller portions throughout the day, or graze, rather than "pig out" at one meal, your body is better able to maintain constant blood sugar levels. When you have low blood sugar, the couch looks awfully good. But since every time you eat your body releases blood sugar from food, if you eat small amounts of superfoods frequently, you'll get a steady stream of blood sugar and feel more like being on the move. Good–bye blood sugar "crashes" and hello *you-on-the-go*. Now imagine what happens if you take the other route and eat big plates only once or twice a day. Your energy will go way up–and then ka–boom, way down. This kind of blood sugar roller coaster is especially hazardous for folks who suffer from insulin–related conditions like diabetes.

Yo! Blood sugar! Respect!
You help the body maintain energy throughout the whole day.

BOOST IN METABOLISM: You want your metabolism to keep churning at a steady pace because that's what digests your food. If you eat a little several times during your cleanse day, your metabolism will keep on truckin'. Turn it around and only eat a couple of whopping meals, after your metabolism is done digesting, there will be lots of time left over when it's just hanging out and idling. The result? Gulp. Packing on the pounds.

BALANCE NUTRIENTS: Research shows people who eat several smaller meals through the day, tend to choose a variety of healthier foods at each meal and get a more balanced diet of fruits, vegetables, fiber, nuts, seeds, and grains. Once you start doing this (if you're not doing it already) you'll see for yourself.

Nutrients – What's That All About?

Heaven knows we've heard the word *nutrient* a million times. Still, there's a good chance most of us know they're good for us but aren't sure exactly what they are, or how they work. On one level that's okay, but sometimes getting a deeper understanding helps to keep us on track.

Simply put, foods and drinks are made up of a range of substances called nutrients. Our bodies utilize them for growth, maintenance of healthy tissues, energy, and to ward off disease. Good nutrition also helps us to think clearly and stay on an even keel. Maybe you know all this, but did you also know that nutrients fall into two main categories:

MACRONUTRIENTS: Since "macro" means large, macronutrients are nutrients needed in large amounts. The majority of our diets are made up of macronutrients that help to supply our body with energy. They include:

- Carbohydrates
- Proteins (including essential amino acids)
- Fats or lipids (including essential fatty acids)
- Water

MICRONUTRIENTS: These are substances we absolutely have to get in tiny amounts from our diet. Why? The answer is our body doesn't make them, or if it does, it can't make them fast enough.

Micronutrients include:
- Vitamins
- Minerals

Superfoods Rock with Micro– *and* Macronutrients

It makes sense that the National Cancer Institute has a campaign to get people to eat five to nine servings of nutritious fruits and vegetables a day. The reason is simple: A diet high in superfoods may prevent or cure a wide range of ailments, including breast cancer, cancer of the colon, esophagus, stomach, lungs, and ovaries, and rectum cancer, as well as asthma, heart disease, and various allergies.

Still have doubts? Maybe this will convince you. For years, epidemiological studies that compare diseases and diets in large populations of people, including those in Africa, China, the Mediterranean, and Russia have shown that folks in countries where the diet consists mostly of fruits and vegetables (making it high in both carbohydrates and fiber) don't suffer with the diseases that afflict North Americans.

During more than 30 years of study, British researchers working in Africa didn't find a single case of such common ailments as diverticulitis, hernia, colon cancer, or prostate cancer. The only reason that they could attribute to the lack of these diseases: differences in diet.

Juicing

But how do you get crazy–busy–sometimes–lazy Americans to eat the recommended daily allowance of fruits and veggies? One answer is juicing! It's not only fairly quick to prepare and easy to eat on the run, but juicing also locks in nutritional freshness. That's because when you eat cooked foods, whether it's grains, fruits, or vegetables, if the food is heated at temperatures above 114°F, healthy enzymes can be destroyed. Since fruits and vegetables are juiced raw, the enzymes are still viable when you drink the juice.

Plus, juicing removes the indigestible fiber but keeps in the digestible kind. These nutrients are available to the body in much larger quantities than if the piece of fruit or vegetable was eaten whole. For example, because many of the nutrients are trapped in the fiber, when you eat a raw carrot, you're only able to assimilate about 1 percent of the available beta–carotene. When a carrot is juiced and the indigestible fiber is removed, nearly 100 percent of the beta–carotene can be assimilated. And yes, juicing can help you lose weight, too.

Tips for Easy Juicing

CLEAN THE PRODUCE: Unwashed fruits and veggies can be contaminated with bacteria so this is an important step in the juicing process. This is true even if it's organic.

SAVE TIME: Prepare your fruits and veggies the night before if you plan on making a morning juice by selecting the ingredients for your juice, washing the produce, placing them in a storage container in the fridge, and assembling the juicer in your kitchen so it's ready to go.

STORE: Juice will keep for 24 to 48 hours in the fridge. But don't forget about it. The max time is 72 hours. If you're traveling, transport your juice in a cooler.

TOP IT OFF: Fill juice to the top of your preferred container to prevent oxygen from getting in, which can deplete the nutrients.

FREEZE: Good news! Freezing is also an option, but only do it right after juicing. Thaw the juice in the fridge.

Must You Buy a Juicer?

Up to you. Most of the recipes offered in the Two-Day Superfood Cleanse require a juicer. If you don't already own a juicer, according to *Consumer Reports*, the type of juice maker you choose depends on the type of juice you like to drink. If you plan to make only citrus juice, then a juicer is the way to go. But if you plan to make your own carrot or vegetable juice, then an extractor is the better choice. In any case, if you've never used or owned a juicer or extractor, don't start off spending a fortune on the top-of-the-line deluxe model. Opt for the mid- or low-end range; use it for a while, and then decide if you want to make juicing a part of your everyday diet. Lots of folks start off enthusiastically but before long their juicers end up collecting dust on a top shelf.

Preparing Fruits and Vegetables

The following recommendations are made by the FDA so it's wise to follow them. According to the Agency, harmful bacteria that may be in the soil or water where produce grows can come in contact with fruits and vegetables and contaminate them. Fresh produce may also become contaminated after it is harvested, such as during preparation or storage. Eating contaminated produce (or fruit and vegetable juices made from contaminated produce) can lead to food-borne illness. Organic produce can also be contaminated.

- When preparing any fresh produce, begin with clean hands. Wash your hands for at least 20 seconds with soap and warm water *before* and *after* preparation.

- Cut away any damaged or bruised areas on fresh fruits and vegetables before preparing and/or eating. Produce that looks rotten should be discarded.

- Wash all produce thoroughly under running water before eating, cutting, or cooking. This includes produce grown conventionally or organically at home, or purchased from a grocery store or farmer's market. Washing fruits and vegetables with soap or detergent or using commercial produce washes is not recommended.

- Even if you plan to peel the produce before eating, it is still important to wash it first so dirt and bacteria aren't transferred from the knife onto the fruit or vegetable. If you're a visual type, the FDA has a poster called "Wash Fruits and Vegetables" available that you can print and display to remember to wash your produce before eating.

- Scrub firm produce such as melons and cucumbers with a clean produce brush.

- Dry produce with a clean cloth towel or paper towel to further reduce bacteria that may be present.

Store It Right

Store perishable fresh fruits and vegetables (like strawberries, herbs, watercress, and mushrooms) in a clean refrigerator at a temperature of 40°F or below. If you're not sure whether an item should be refrigerated to maintain quality, ask your grocer.

Refrigerate all produce that is purchased precut or peeled to maintain both quality and safety.

Keep your refrigerator set at 40°F or below. Use a fridge thermometer to check!

How Do You Know if Food Is Really Organic?

The U.S. Department of Agriculture (USDA) will say so. Organic produce is grown without using most conventional pesticides, fertilizers made with synthetic ingredients, or sewage sludge, bioengineering, or ionizing radiation. Before a product can be labeled "organic," a government-approved certifier inspects the farm where the food is grown to make sure the farmer meets the USDA's organic standards. Companies that handle or process organic food before it reaches the supermarket or restaurant must be certified, too.

What About My Local Farmer's Market?

Food from the farmer's market will be fresh, but there's no guarantee of its organic status. Small local farmers often use organic methods but then can't afford to become certified organic through the USDA. It's a great idea to visit a farmer's market and talk with the farmers. Find out how they grow their fruits and vegetables. You can even ask for a farm tour. Generally local food means food is grown close to home. During certain times of the year, the farmer's market can offer a huge bounty of healthy foods while benefiting your budget big time.

More Ways to Stay Healthy and Save $$$

SHARE IN A COMMUNITY-SUPPORTED AGRICULTURE PROGRAM (CSA): This means you pay a portion of a local farm's operating expenses. In return, you receive weekly cartons of fresh fruits and vegetables in the upcoming harvest. Most shares in a CSA cost about $300 to $400 upfront for a 24- to 26-week growing season. Many CSA programs accept weekly or monthly payments, and you may be able to buy a half-share rather than a whole share. And don't think just because you live in a city you can't join a CSA. Look on the web for a CSA near you.

GO CO-OP: This is a member-owned business that provides groceries and other products to its members at a discount. Lots of products for sale in co-ops are organic and much of the produce comes from local family farms. Joining a co-op is often as easy as signing up and paying some dues. Co-op members that volunteer to work may get additional discounts on products they buy.

JOIN A BUYING CLUB: It's a terrific way to get organic food inexpensively. In a buying club, you may be able to get 30 to 40 percent off the retail price. Buying-club members purchase food and other organic products in bulk and then split the stash.

BUY IN BULK: It doesn't matter whether you're shopping in your natural food store or supermarket, buying in bulk can save money. Bulk products include superfood beans, grains, nuts, and seeds. Just be certain you have a cool, dry place to store your dry goods. But don't be tempted to buy in bulk if you don't think you'll eat all your stash.

BE FLEXIBLE: To grab a good deal on organic food you need to be a flexible flier. Even if you're shopping with a list of superfoods, buy a good bargain when you see one. For example, choose among three superfood vegetables on your shopping list and see if anything is on "special." Do the same for your fruits, nuts, seeds, and grains.

Faith and prayer are the vitamins of the soul; man cannot live in health without them.

~ Mahalia Jackson

Caution: Supplements

Can vitamin and mineral supplements be bad for your health? Sometimes. It's ironic because the root of the word vitamin is *vita*, which in Latin means "life." And certainly, in order to live we need vitamins to convert our food into energy. But the question is how many do we need, or more importantly, can't we get enough vitamins and minerals from superfoods? The answer is yes! You get the required amount of vitamins and minerals from superfoods. That's what they're all about.

But manufacturers of vitamin and mineral supplements argue that most diets don't have enough and we need to take pills to make up for our lack of nutrients. But here's the danger: Research shows that large quantities of supplemental vitamins and minerals may do more harm than good.

Let's look at these facts: In a study published in the *New England Journal of Medicine*, 29,000 Finnish men, all smokers, had been given daily vitamin E, beta–carotene, both, or a placebo. The study found that those who had taken beta–carotene for five to eight years were more likely to die from lung cancer or heart disease than those who hadn't taken supplements. In another study on vitamin supplements, 18,000 people who were at an increased risk of lung cancer because of asbestos exposure or smoking received a combination of vitamin A and beta–carotene, or a placebo. Scientists halted the study. Why? They discovered that the risk of death from lung cancer for those who took the vitamins was 46 percent higher. Another review of 14 randomized trials found that the supplemental vitamins

A, C, E and beta-carotene, and a mineral, selenium, taken to prevent intestinal cancers, actually increased mortality.

Vitamin E supplements seem to be particularly toxic. A review, published in the *Annals of Internal Medicine*, found that in 19 trials of nearly 136,000 people, supplemental vitamin E increased mortality. And a study of people with vascular disease or diabetes found that vitamin E increased their risk of heart failure. A study just a couple of years ago published in the *Journal of the American Medical Association* made a connection between vitamin E supplements and an increased risk of prostate cancer.

Scientists suspect the reason for supplemental toxicity might simply be a matter of too much of a good thing. Yes, folks who eat more antioxidant-packed superfood fruits and vegetables have a lower incidence of cancer and heart disease and live longer. Doesn't it reason that even more would be even better? Not so fast. When people take large doses of antioxidants in the form of supplemental vitamins, the balance between free radical production and destruction might tip too much in one direction, causing an unnatural state where the immune system is less able to kill harmful invaders.

What's the best advice? Stick to a superfood diet and chuck those bottled supplements. For true life.

If you do take supplements, be sure to ask your doctor about possible side effects and interactions with any medications you take.

Exceptions

Women who may become pregnant should get 400 micrograms a day of folic acid from fortified foods or supplements, in addition to eating foods that naturally contain folate. Women who are pregnant should take a prenatal vitamin that includes iron or a separate iron supplement. Adults age 50 or older should eat foods fortified with vitamin B12, such as fortified cereals, or take a multivitamin that contains B12 or a separate B12 supplement.

If you have a medical condition that affects how your body absorbs or uses nutrients, such as chronic diarrhea, food allergies, food intolerance, or a disease of the liver, gallbladder, intestines, or pancreas, talk to your doctor about taking the correct supplements.

If you have had surgery on your digestive tract and are not able to digest and absorb nutrients properly, check with your doctor before taking any supplements.

Quiz
Are You Ready for the Two-Day Superfood Cleanse?

Some of us are primed at the pump, right here and right now, to experience the Superfood Cleanse, while others may not be as ready to put our pedal to the metal. Although certain advocates of cleansing might suggest you need to "just do it" regardless of what else is swirling around in your life, I'm not that person. You first need to be ready to commit to making healthy adjustments in your life and then set the stage for change. No worries! No matter where you stand on the scale, with simple preparations you'll be ready to begin your cleansing adventure.

Choose either A, B, or C. Then total your score and read the analysis.

1. As I envision going on the Superfood Cleanse, I see that:
   a. I'll have to give up an awful lot.
   b. Sure, I'll have to pass on junk food, but the rewards will make up for what I'll miss.
   c. I'm looking forward to moving toward an even healthier diet.

2. When I think about beginning any project now, I feel:

    a. Overwhelmed. There's already a crisis situation in my life I'm dealing with.

    b. A little anxious. I'll have to balance my family, work, and relationship responsibilities.

    c. Excited! It couldn't be a better time!

3. Juicing seems like:

    a. A luxury. I'm already so busy.

    b. A manageable idea. I'll just have to schedule in time for the food prep.

    c. A snap. I already do it.

4. When it comes to seeing projects to the end, I:

    a. Am easily distracted.

    b. Will do it, but it takes me time.

    c. Am a deadline fanatic.

5. When it comes to learning new recipes, I:

    a. Am not that into it since I don't like to try new foods.

    b. Prefer to try unfamiliar dishes at restaurants, but I'll give it a whirl.

    c. Love to cook!

6. I'm looking for a new approach to dieting because:

    a. My partner (or doctor) keeps getting on my case about being too heavy and I need to try something.

    b. I'm done with fad diets. I want to make changes that will help me to lose weight and keep me healthy for life.

    c. Research shows it's a nutritionally sound approach.

7. I imagine I'll lose:

    a. A lot of weight very quickly.

    b. A few pounds a week.

    c. About one pound a week.

8. Have I resolved emotional issues connected to my eating habits and weight?

   a. Not really.

   b. I'm getting there.

   c. I've dealt with the deep issues.

9. Do you have people in your life who support your goals?

   a. My partner, but mostly I like to do things on my own.

   b. One best buddy I know I can count on and then a wide circle of less close companions.

   c. A tight circle of supportive friends who want the best for me.

10. My stress level is:

   a. Off the charts.

   b. Somewhere in the middle.

   c. I'm coasting.

Mostly A's: Don't Start Your Superfood Cleanse Tomorrow!

It's not that you don't have what it takes, but it seems like your life right now is pretty stressful. Devoting yourself to a Superfood Cleanse isn't really a big deal, but if you're not in the right frame of mind, it can feel more challenging than it needs to be. You don't want to set yourself up to fail. Right? So try to relax, take a deep breath, and wait just two weeks before experiencing the cleanse. By starting off slowly and accomplishing small goals, you may see that you have everything it takes to succeed in your cleansing and diet efforts. In the meantime, here's what you can do to prepare:

- Write down a schedule that includes time to shop and prepare meals. If it needs to be reworked, use this waiting period to make changes in your lifestyle. This might mean clearing out responsibilities that no longer serve you or making better use of downtime.

- Meditate: Try sitting comfortably in a quiet place for just 15 minutes a day. When thoughts come up (and they will) just let them pass like clouds in the sky. Countless studies show regular meditation reduces stress – big time.

- Rally some support: Make sure your partner or closest friends are willing to help you stick to your Superfood Cleanse. Be aware of any folks who might sabotage your cleanse and schedule meetings with them on non-cleansing days.

- Practice reducing your intake of sugar, caffeine, alcohol, or processed foods.

Mostly B's: You're Ready to Superfood Cleanse on Nonconsecutive Days

Now is as good a time as any to enjoy the Two-Day Superfood Cleanse and the best way for you to do it – until you get your food chops sharpened – is to enjoy cleansing on non-consecutive days. It will be much easier for you to stick to the plan if you give yourself time between Superfood Cleanse days to enjoy your favorite meals. You'll be less likely to feel as if you're depriving yourself. Eventually, your taste buds will go through a transformation and you'll actually crave nutritious superfoods. If you want to bump up your cleansing power, these tips will help:

- Try one new recipe on a Sunday afternoon when you have more time.

- Put some superfoods you usually don't eat into your non-cleansing diet days when there's no calorie limit.

- Visit farmer's markets, browse a health food store or the organic section of your supermarket, and familiarize yourself with superfoods. Also, buy some products in bulk.

- Vow to put down your fork on non–cleanse days once you're feeling satiated. No more "pigging out"!

Mostly C's: You're Ready for an Even Deeper Detox—Go for a Two-Day Cleanse

Many of these superfoods are already part of your regular diet. Compared to most Americans, you live a healthy lifestyle by exercising regularly, keeping stress at bay, and paying attention to subtle signs when your body isn't functioning 100 percent. Plus, you have a great support system. All these factors make you the ideal candidate to increase your cleansing capabilities by experiencing the diet on two consecutive days. By doing so you'll give your body's organs the opportunity to enjoy a deeper, more substantial detoxification and the results will be profound. To further ease into a two–day consecutive cleanse:

- Look at your monthly calendar and choose the days that work best for you. Weekends are often an excellent time to engage in consecutive–day cleansing.

- Go deeper. If you already meditate, increase the time. The same goes for any yoga, qigong, or tai chi practices. If you don't engage in any of these forms, try at least one.

- Pay attention to changes. Since you're already on the right track, keep a journal to record how you're feeling both physically and emotionally. For you the changes may be more subtle, but definitely worth noting.

- Laugh! Admit it. Sometimes you take life a bit too seriously. If you need some encouragement to lighten up, consider research that shows the therapeutic benefits of laughing. Watch a funny movie, read a humorous book, or tickle someone and expect the same in return. No joke.

4
Building Willpower

The most important thing in life is to stop saying "I wish"
and start saying "I will."

~ *Charles Dickens*

During your first few tries at Superfood Cleanse days you may
find yourself sitting on the fence or you might be totally gung-
ho and already exuberant about climbing to new heights of
wellness. No matter what your level of enthusiasm, what will
ultimately determine whether you stay with the plan or not is
a firm commitment coupled with mighty willpower. Does that
mean on some level it's out of your control? Hardly! Scientists
have found there are several strategies you can use to develop
these factors. Think of your willpower as a muscle. The more
you exercise it, the stronger it becomes.

What's more, there's solid evidence that the simpler you make your diet, the more chance you'll have to meet success. The Two-Day Superfood Cleanse does just that by reminding you that the big so-called secret to diet loss doesn't exist. Losing weight can be reduced to this simple mantra: *calories in, calories out*. Again, if you eat fewer calories than you burn, you'll lose weight. If you make those calories superfoods that are high in nutrients, you'll reap even more benefits than just dropping pounds; you'll be guaranteed all-around health, wellness, and inner and outer beauty.

Biggest Saboteurs

Be prepared to fight those nasty forces that might dull your enthusiasm by recognizing a good attitude's enemies. Here they are:

THINKING ALL HEALTH FOODS ARE LOW-CALORIE: Even though every one of the superfoods offered in this cleanse are amazingly good for your well-being, they're not all low-calorie. While whole grains and nuts are superstars, they might also be high in calories and fat. What to do? Definitely enjoy these calorie-rich super healthy foods, but ration them out. Don't even think about binging on these calorie-packed morsels.

LOSING SLEEP: It's not uncommon to feel a surge of energy when your body is fueled by superfoods; if you feel this way, use your new bounce to enjoy life to the limit, exercise like a bunny, finish a project, or begin a new one. But don't do any of these things late in the day. This can keep you awake at night, which is bad news, and there's research linking shorter sleep duration to a higher body mass index (a measure of body fat) and increased hunger and appetite. In addition, if you're tired *and* hungry, you'll be more tempted to down a sugary treat for a midday boost, avoid exercise, and order out rather than prepare a superfood recipe. Watch out for this sabotaging cycle and always aim for seven or eight hours of shut-eye each night.

MISCALCULATING: Quick! How many calories have you eaten today? No idea? Dieticians say calorie ignorance is common and it's fueled by a few factors. First, there's a warped understanding of portion size, so at the beginning of the cleanse, you'll need to measure *everything*. Also, pay attention to a seemingly innocent choice like your juice concoction. You might end up juicing a little extra and think "Oh, I can't waste this!" and then top your glass off *again*. Well, that could be 50 precious calories right there!

OVERESTIMATING CALORIES BURNED: Do you tend to reward yourself with extra food, thinking you've burned it off with exercise? Perhaps you should reconsider. Suppose you go for a 30-minute jog. The University of Maryland Medical Center's "calories burned calculator" estimates that a 150-pound person would burn about 370 calories. But what if you strolled and didn't jog? Add at least 200 back on.

ENVIRONMENTAL TEMPTATION: Do a purge around your house and get rid of all the high-calorie, low-nutrition junk foods in your pantry and refrigerator and substitute them with yummy superfoods. What if coworkers make it a habit of bringing their home-baked muffins to the office or routinely put out bowls of chips or M&Ms on your cleanse day? First of all, thank your lucky stars for such generous colleagues! Second, oh, no! The best strategy is to implore a coworker to go on the same health-kick as you. There's power in numbers.

SAVING UP CALORIES SO YOU CAN EAT JUNK FOOD: You could eat a bag of chips 'til the cows come home, but that's not going to make you feel satiated. Without enough superfood protein, fiber, vitamins, and minerals, you'll be ravenous an hour later and blow your calorie limit. Don't fool yourself.

MEDICATIONS: Some drugs, including antidepressants and beta blockers commonly cause weight gain and they can interfere with your low-calorie program. While treating your primary medical condition is important, you may be able to find a substitute that doesn't increase your weight. Speak with your doctor.

FAMILY AND FRIENDS: Of course, you don't want to break Granny's heart and turn down her gooey pineapple upside-down cake topped with marshmallow fluff, nor do you want to pass on a serving of her triple-fried chicken, so don't visit her during one of your Superfood Cleanse days. The same goes for nights out with friends if they routinely revolve around food-and-drink binges. A report in the *New England Journal of Medicine* found that one's chance of becoming overweight increases by 57 percent if a close friend becomes obese. Try to keep your two chosen days of Superfood Cleanse absolutely sacred, and reschedule nights out on the town with those partying buds.

Six Ways to Pump Up Your Willpower

1 **FOCUS:** According to Kelly McGonigal, PhD, a health psychologist at Stanford University and author of the *The Willpower Instinct*, each time you sit down to meditate you're exercising two crucial parts of your brain that relate to willpower: the prefrontal cortex, which helps you make smart choices, and the anterior cingulate cortex, which helps you be aware of when you make such choices and when you don't. The more you activate these systems, the more powerful they become, so in the future it will feel easier to do the right thing.

2 **USE A TWO-PRONG STRATEGY:** Is it your nature to be a wishful thinker and imagine that if you have the right focus and determination, it's guaranteed you'll evolve into

Jessica Alba's body double? Or are you more of a downer, complaining about how hard it is to resist "real" food when you're out in the world. Well, guess what? Each of these attitudes can help you stay on your cleanse–but only if you embrace them both, *equally*. Surprisingly, according to researchers from New York University in New York City and the University of Hamburg in Germany, embracing both attitudes *at the same time* is the secret to sticking to a particular diet plan. In other words, if you imagine succeeding and then reflect on the obstacles facing you, you'll be more inspired to reach a goal than if you do solely one or the other.

3   **DEVISE PLAN B:** What if you're starving and find yourself standing in front of the candy aisle? Or what if it's the night to go out and celebrate your friend's birthday and oops, you forgot it's also your Superfood Cleanse day? Devising a plan B will help you cope with situations that may undo you. That's what New York University researchers discovered in their study of students who wanted to eat less junk food. When the students thought through tempting scenarios in advance and made "if-then" plans specifying how to overcome these temptations, it was easier for them to stick to their healthy choices.

4   **OFFER A DIFFERENT REWARD:** Our bodies have been hardwired over years of evolution to seek rewards such as food and sex to keep us alive. When the brain identifies a reward, it shifts into a state of intense focus and drive. But you can use that drive to your advantage simply by changing the reward in any given situation. Make the choice: "Do I want to be one step closer to my dream body or not?" It's easier to go after something you want than something you don't want. When temptation strikes, focus on a positive reward that will help you sidestep it. What might that be? How about some yummy goji berries?

5   **RETHINK:** You can kill cravings for sugary delights—*really*—by steering your thoughts away from particularly sweet treats. For example, when you see a red velvet cupcake in the window of a bake shop, don't think about how delicious the frosting must be, but focus instead on its gorgeous decoration. Keep taste out of the equation and you'll be more likely to pass on sweet concoctions.

6   **PRACTICE FORGIVENESS:** You know how to treat your friends and loved ones with kindness and compassion. Why not do the same for yourself? If during a moment of weakness you blew your Superfood Cleanse day by succumbing to temptation, remind yourself it's not the end of the world. There's always tomorrow. Folks who overstep their 600-calorie Superfood Cleanse day and then beat themselves up about it actually eat more because they feel so bad about themselves. Instead, ask yourself: What if a friend were upset that she skipped her diet day? You'd probably tell her one day isn't so bad, and then you'd encourage her to hop back on the wagon right away. Right? If you slip up, try to be as kind and forgiving to yourself.

It's always too early to quit.

~ *Norman Vincent Peale*

How to Make a Commitment

Most of us start off with excellent intentions. But unless we couple our willpower with a strong commitment, we'll constantly be tested and tempted. A commitment offers a deeper purpose to our desire to live a healthier lifestyle. Here are some tips to help bolster your commitment to the Superfood Cleanse:

KNOW YOUR TARGET WEIGHT: Experts say it helps to know how much you need to lose before you begin your cleanse.

Anywhere between 5 and 20 pounds is a reasonable goal. Keep track of your weight loss with a chart. Recognizing the progress you've made also helps firm your commitment.

MATCH YOUR CLEANSE WITH EXERCISE: Studies show that dieters who couple their program with exercise not only tend to lose more weight and keep it off longer, but their minds stay focused on their goals.

KEEP TRACK: You're more likely to stick to a cleanse if you keep track of what you're eating. Studies show putting something in writing cements commitment.

DON'T BE IN A HURRY: Take your time and don't expect drastic results immediately. If you've had a lifetime of unhealthy eating or it took you two years to put that weight on, it's not going to be gone in two weeks. Be kind and remind yourself that you're doing the best that you can. Any change for the better is great, so reward your efforts regularly maybe with a relaxing massage or a night out dancing.

USE YOUR IMAGINATION: Studies show our bodies are capable of responding to virtual situations in the same way they respond to real ones. In one study, participants were asked to watch a movie, and a bowl of chocolate candy was placed nearby. One group was told to imagine they had decided to eat as much as they wanted, a second group was told to imagine they had decided to eat none, and a third group was told to imagine they'd decided to eat them later on. The first group did indeed eat more than the other two groups. But when given the opportunity to eat candy later, those who imagined they would delay eating the candy actually ate significantly less than the other two groups. They even reported having less desire for candy when queried through e-mail on the following day.

PUT THOUGHTS IN YOUR HEAD: How do you avoid thinking about going off your cleanse? Well, train yourself to think about something else: For example, every time you think about eating a slice of pizza, think about eating a yummy superfood instead. This will put you in the driver's seat of your thoughts.

LEARN TO CONTROL STRESS HORMONES: The stress hormone cortisol boosts cravings, especially for carbs, because carbs physiologically lower cortisol levels. But the downside of dealing with stress this way is that, in the long run, you risk diabetes, cardiovascular disease, and weight gain. Every time you respond to cortisol surges through unhealthy means, you strengthen those habits. This practically guarantees that under times of stress, you'll fall back on these unhealthy habits. Try responding to mild stressors with healthier choices, such as listening to calming music or visualizing calming scenes.

BE TRUE TO YOURSELF: It takes an enormous amount of effort to suppress your normal personality, preferences, and behaviors. Not surprisingly, doing so depletes commitment and willpower. Psychologists say folks who exert this kind of self–control in order to please others are more easily depleted than people who hold true to their own internal goals and desires. When it comes to willpower and commitment, people–pleasers may find themselves at a disadvantage compared to those who are secure and comfortable with themselves.

UNDERSTAND YOURSELF: To be successful, it's essential to understand *why* you want to be on the cleanse. Before you begin, ask yourself (and answer honestly):

- Am I really ready to do this?
- Is my motivation coming from within?
- Can I deal with occasional setbacks or lack of progress?
- Can I fully focus on the cleanse? (If you're in the midst of a crisis, it's probably better to resolve it first.)

Ten Steps to Positive Thinking

1 **OWN UP TO IT:** Just like everyone else, you experience more than 50,000 thoughts each day. And these thoughts are yours alone. Taking responsibility for what you're thinking and feeling is the first step in gaining the ability to change your thinking patterns.

2 **CREATE A STRATEGY:** As you know, there's a lot of negative thinking out there, so you'll need to develop ways you can work around it. It may seem like an overwhelming project, but you can make it simple. One thing you can do is to identify and record your negative thoughts each day, and then take time to reflect on why you had those thoughts and how you can improve them. By noting your triggers and reactions during these trying, stressful times, you'll have something concrete to work with to change for the better.

3 **KISS BLACK AND WHITE THINKING GOOD-BYE:** Because if you hold onto it, everything you encounter *is* or it *isn't*—there are no shades of gray. Try embracing the subtleties in life. Instead of thinking in terms of two outcomes, one positive and one negative, make a list of all of the outcomes in between. Considering the subtleties in any situation will help you see that it's almost never the end of the world. Even when you feel like your back is pushed up against the wall, there's always a step to take to lead you away.

4 **AVOID CATASTROPHIZING:** This is when you can't think of anything without assuming it's all going to end in

doom and gloom. Be practical. Think of the likelihood of something completely devastating happening. For example, if you fall into a negative panic every time a loved one is on an airplane, remember that a person has a better chance of dying by getting hit over the head with a falling brick than in a plane crash. When it comes to catastrophic thinking relating to your cleanse it goes like this: I ate 800 instead of 600 calories today and now all the hard work I've done is ruined. I'll never be able to make up for it. My body is a mess! Sounds silly, right?

5   **GET RID OF THE CRYSTAL BALL:** If you spend your time as a fortune teller deciding the future according to what you've experienced in the past, you'll be convinced that you're never going to change your eating habits. If you hear yourself saying "Why shouldn't I fail, I have all the other times," there's no room for positive thinking to lead you to a positive outcome. Instead, learn to take things on a case-by-case basis.

6   **TAKE YOUR TIME:** Developing a positive outlook means developing a skill. Even though none of us are born thinking negatively, it happens over time as we mirror the world around us. As with any skill, a can-do attitude takes mastery. It also requires dedication and gentle reminders about not falling back into negative thinking. So say positive things about yourself, regularly. How you communicate to yourself affects your thinking and your emotions, as well as your self-esteem.

7   **TRY NEW THINGS:** A wide variety of life experiences can do wonders for sticking to a cleanse. It may seem unrelated, but stepping out of your comfort zone affects everything, including how you take care of your body. Something as simple as trying a new superfood recipe can lead to the

discovery of new tastes and different sensations, along with the release of negative prior impressions.

8 **ENJOY YOUR CREATIVE SIDE:** If you haven't had a chance to explore your creative side, now's the time. Taking the time to be artistic and to work with your hands or explore your most original thoughts can do wonders for your power to think outside the box and to therefore think positively. Even if you don't think you're naturally inclined toward creativity, there are a number of ways you can express yourself to become more positive.

9 **SURROUND YOURSELF WITH UPBEAT PEOPLE:** Positivity is infectious. On the flip side, so is negativity. That's why if you want to be infected by optimism, you need to associate with folks who see the glass as half full. Make it a point to avoid folks who suck your energy and motivation. If you absolutely can't avoid them, keep the time you spend together brief.

10 **HAVE FUN!:** Okay, it's a cliché but it's said often for good reason – people who seek a bit of regular fun in their lives tend to be happier and more positive because it isn't all drudgery and never-ending monotony. Fun breaks up the hard work and challenges. Plug let-loose time into your schedule. If you're a stressed-out workaholic with no opportunity for fun, you'll be much more likely to think negatively.

What about Food Cravings?

Yeah. Yeah. Yeah. Willpower. Commitment. Positive thinking. But what about when you're absolutely dying for a bag of chips, a chewy candy bar, or a mocha? We've all been there. Cravings can be so intense they consume our every thought. To say they're tough to shake is like saying Mt. Everest is just a hill. It turns out one of the most effective strategies to dealing with a craving is to understand what's triggering it.

That's where Alan R. Hirsch, MD, head of the Smell & Taste Treatment and Research Foundation in Chicago and the author of *What Flavor Is Your Personality?* comes in. He's studied the cravings of more than 18,000 people for over 25 years and has come to some conclusions about why we yearn for certain foods.

SALTY: Studies have shown that women who eat low-calcium diets want salty foods more than those who have enough calcium in their bodies. That's because sodium temporarily increases calcium levels in the blood, which tricks the body into thinking the problem is solved. Or, it might be a mineral imbalance. Researchers have also found that a lack of potassium, calcium, and iron causes animal test subjects to pig out on table salt.

CHOCOLATE: This confection stimulates the release of serotonin, the feel-good brain chemical. Think of it as an antidepressant in dessert form. So if you're feeling blue, you'll be more likely to crave a chocolate treat.

SPICY: There's been research pointing to the premise that people can become addicted to spicy food's rush. If you love the taste of hot sauce, it may be because hot foods raise blood pressure, accelerate heart rate, and increase breathing rate. You thrill seeker!

SWEET: This might mean you're feeling low on energy. The body absorbs refined sugars faster than any other type of food, offering you immediate fuel. But as most of us know by now, after soaring comes the dull thump of a crash.

Looking Ahead

In the next chapter you'll be given plenty of simple recipes to choose from during your Superfood Cleanse days. Although there are numerous delicious and easy options, you might be tempted to slip back into eating unhealthy foods. The inner force that can help you stick to your goal may be hidden even from yourself. This quick test may help you uncover it.

Quiz
What Gives You a Winning Edge?

1. If you realized you'd been overcharged $5 after returning home from the supermarket, you'd:

   a. Seek a refund the next time you went there.

   b. Set the receipt aside, but probably forget about it.

   c. Drive back right away.

2. If the book you were reading became boring in the middle, you'd probably:

   a. Finish it anyway.

   b. Skip to the good parts.

   c. Move on to something you enjoy.

3. When the cell phone rings, you usually:

   a. Check to see who it is before answering, then decide.

   b. Let it go to voicemail. If it's so important, there's text.

   c. Answer it right away.

4. If you won a lot of money, you'd spend it on:

   a. An investment opportunity.

   b. A dream home or car.

   c. Making a fantasy come true, like a five-star trip or piece of jewelry.

5. **If you were involved in a theater production, the job you'd most want is:**
   a. *Director.*
   b. *Stage manager.*
   c. *Lead actor.*

6. **On the second day of the Superfood Cleanse, someone offers you a fabulous dessert. You would most likely:**
   a. *Politely decline.*
   b. *Take a nibble.*
   c. *Use it solely for your 600-calorie limit.*

7. **If you reach a two-way stop sign at the same time as another driver, you'd:**
   a. *Wait and let the other car go.*
   b. *Make eye contact to size up who should move first.*
   c. *Try to go first.*

Mostly A's: Your Winning Edge Is Willpower

Once you decide on a course of action, you stick with it and let nothing get in your way. That's because you see yourself as the master of your own destiny. Natural willpower is fueled by the dominant personality traits restraint, resolve, and discipline. You've got plenty of all three, so temptation has no power over you.

Mostly B's: Your Winning Edge Is Flexibility

If you hit a detour, you don't feel frustrated; you just try to figure out how to make the alternate route work for you. Naturally open-minded, you have a knack for considering all points of view before reaching a decision. This "big picture" approach also helps you adapt to any new situation or unplanned obstacle with ease. Even if a superfood option isn't available in the moment, you know how to make a sensible substitution without blowing your Superfood Cleanse completely.

Mostly C's: Your Winning Edge Is Passion

No matter what you take on, you bring your whole heart and soul to it, making it your new "cause." For you, if there isn't a flame burning deep inside, there's no reason to get involved with a project – and that goes for dieting and cleansing. Your drive to leave your mark makes you positively unstoppable. Eager to try new things, your boundless spirit keeps you moving forward until you reach your weight loss and wellness goals.

Superfood Recipes

Food is an important part of a balanced diet.
~ Fran Lebowitz

Are your taste buds dreading the 600-calorie cleanse days? Well, give that anxious critic a tongue lashing. Tell it you won't have to choose between yummy dishes and good-for-you meals because these recipes are both: nutritious *and* delicious.

On the following pages you'll be offered lots of tantalizing and simple-to-make juices and dishes all created with the top fresh superfoods. Although some of the offerings may be new and even strange to your palate, give them a chance. Opening up to new experiences is also part of the Superfood Cleanse.

Hint: Use your math smarts or your phone's calculator to add calories throughout your cleanse day. Did I mention you're on a *low-calorie* cleanse? You'll also need to be strict about portion size for the same reason. Many recipes are for two servings or more, so you'll need to divide the dish appropriately and share with others or savor the leftovers the following day.

A Word about Freshness

The nutritional value of most fruits and vegetables deteriorates over a pretty short period of time, usually between 24 hours and three days. It's a good rule not to store any of these foods for too long before using them. Refrigeration helps to hold in more of the nutrients; the exception is citrus fruits, which need to be kept at room temperature. Avocados ripen at room temperature, but then they should be put in the fridge immediately. Store nuts, seeds, and grains in airtight containers and then in a dry, dark place.

Don't be tempted to prepare any recipes with bruised or blemished fruits or vegetables. They not only won't taste as good, but they'll likely be lacking in nutrients.

Juices

If you're going to be enjoying juices as part of your cleanse (and this is only one option), you'll need a juicer. There are lots of different models available from different manufacturers, but there are basically only two types:

CENTRIFUGAL JUICER: This less expensive option spins the fruit or vegetable around a serrated blade and strains the juice through a filter. It either retains the pulp or ejects it into another container. Washing and maintaining this juicer takes time.

MASTICATING JUICER: This is a larger and heavier machine and, not surprisingly, costs more. It works by crushing ingredients between rollers and pushing them through a wire mesh. This mechanism means more juice and drier leftover pulp. Opt for a juicer with a spout. That way the juice goes directly into your glass rather than into a jug that's tough to keep clean.

A blender is an option if you're drinking smoothies exclusively and don't need to press or grind vegetables.

Get Preppie

The secret to truly great juicing is in the preparation. Immediately before using, wash your organic fruits and vegetables thoroughly under cold running water and then rub off any dirt. If your ingredients aren't organic, you'll need to use a bristled brush to scrub them. Grapefruits, kiwis, and coconuts should be peeled but apples, sweet potatoes, and radishes need not be.

Hint:
Be sure you fully juice your leafy vegetables like spinach and watercress by wrapping each leaf around a chunk of fruit or other veggies.

Lemons Love You

You'll notice that many of these recipes contain lemons. Although technically not considered a superfood, lemons can make drinks and solid foods taste just a little richer, fuller, and tangier. They're also full of health benefits. Lemons have strong antibacterial, antiviral, and immune-boosting powers, and they make an excellent weight-loss aid because they help both with digestion and liver cleansing. These yellow lovelies also contain citric acid, calcium, magnesium, vitamin C, bioflavonoids, pectin, and limonene, which promote immunity and fight infection.

1 MEDIUM LEMON: 17 calories

Juice Recipes

Sour Apple

SERVES: 2 | CALORIES: 87 per serving

2 apples, cut into wedges
½ lemon, peeled and quartered
1 lime, peeled and quartered

Press the chunks of fruit through a juicer.

Apple Grape Love

SERVES: 2 | CALORIES: 115 per serving

2 apples, cut into wedges
25 seedless grapes

Press alternate fruits through the juicer.

Cabbage Currant Concoction

SERVES: 2 | CALORIES: 196 per serving

½ medium cabbage, leaves separated and core chopped into chunks
3 large carrots
12 black currants

While running the cabbage and carrot chunks through a juicer, alternate with black currants.

Simple Grapefruit Sip

SERVES: 1 | CALORIES: 41

½ grapefruit peeled and torn into segments

Pass the segments through a juicer.

Carrot and Flax Fantastico

SERVES: 1 | CALORIES: 126

2 large carrots, chopped
2 cloves garlic, chopped
½ tablespoon flaxseed oil

Alternate passing the carrots and garlic through the juicer. Stir in the oil and drink immediately.

Watercress Wonder

SERVES: 2 | CALORIES: 162 per serving

1 bunch watercress
4 medium apples, cut into wedges
½ lemon, cut into wedges

Wrap watercress around apples slices and pass through a juicer. Squeeze the lemon wedges into the juice.

Tangy Tomato

SERVES: 1 | CALORIES: 61

2 large tomatoes, cut into wedges
1 lemon, peeled and quartered

Pass alternating chunks of tomato and lemon through a juicer. Drink immediately.

Goji Apple Grape Gusher

SERVES: 2 | CALORIES: 114 per serving

2 apples, cut into wedges
15 seedless grapes
10 goji berries

Press alternate chunks of apple and grapes through a juicer. Top with goji berries. Drink immediately.

Watercress and Tomato Tango

SERVES: 1 | CALORIES: 58

½ bunch watercress
2½ large tomatoes, cut into wedges

Wrap watercress around the tomato chunks and pass through a juicer. Stir and drink immediately.

Watermelon Refresher

SERVES: 2 | CALORIES: 350 per serving

½ (16-pound) watermelon peeled, seeded, and chopped into chunks

Pass the watermelon chunks through a juicer. Stir and drink immediately.

Green Dream

SERVES: 2 | CALORIES: 241 per serving

1 cup fresh spinach leaves
10 seedless grapes
½ medium avocado, peeled and pitted
1 apple, cut into wedges
1 cup ice

Pass the spinach leaves, grapes, avocado, apple, and ice through a juicer.

Orange You Green

SERVES: 2 | CALORIES: 223 per serving

1 cup fresh spinach leaves
2 oranges, peeled and cut into segments
3 kiwis, peeled and cut into chunks

Wrap the spinach leaves around orange and kiwi pieces. Press through a juicer.

Orange Coconut

SERVES: 2 | CALORIES: 202 per serving

2 oranges, peeled and cut into segments
1 fresh coconut, broken in half, flesh scraped out

Press alternate chunks of fruit through a juicer. Stir and drink immediately.

Kiwi Orange Carrot Delight

SERVES: 1 | CALORIES: 65

1 orange, peeled and cut into segments
1 kiwi, peeled and chopped into chunks
1 large carrot, chopped into chunks

Alternate passing fruit pieces through a juicer. Shake and drink immediately.

Solid Food

Nuts

Hot Almonds

SERVES: 2 | CALORIES: 75 per serving

1½ cups raw unblanched almonds
1½ tablespoons honey
½ teaspoon chili powder
¼ teaspoon salt

Toast the almonds in a nonstick skillet over medium heat for 5 minutes until lightly toasted, shaking the pan often. Then combine the rest of the ingredients in a 2–cup microwave–safe cup and microwave on high for 30 seconds. Add the honey mixture to the pan with the almonds and cook for 2 more minutes. To avoid sticking or burning, stir constantly. Spread the almonds on a baking sheet lined with parchment paper and let it stand for at least 15 minutes until cool. Store in an airtight container for up to a week.

Spinach with Lemon and Pine Nuts
SERVES: 2 | CALORIES: 142 per serving

1 tablespoon extra-virgin olive oil
juice of ½ lemon
¼ teaspoon dried thyme
1 (9-ounce) bag fresh baby spinach
2 tablespoons pine nuts
salt

In a small bowl, whisk together the olive oil, lemon juice, and thyme. Set aside. Meanwhile place a steamer basket in a large saucepan over a couple inches of water. Add the spinach to the steamer basket, cover the pan, and turn the heat to medium-high. Cook until the spinach just wilts, 3 to 4 minutes. Place spinach in a bowl and toss with the lemon–oil dressing. Add the pine nuts and season with salt to taste.

Amazing Apple and Walnut Salad
SERVES: 6 (1 cup each) | CALORIES: 155 per serving

2 cups torn red leaf lettuce
½ large red apple, chopped
½ large green apple, chopped
¼ cup chopped walnuts, toasted
⅓ cup thinly sliced red onion
⅓ cup dried goji berries
juice of ½ lemon
salt and pepper

In a salad bowl, toss together all the ingredients except the lemon juice. Spritz the lemon over the salad. Season with salt and pepper to taste. Serve immediately.

Brazil Nut Faux Cheese Treat

SERVES: 6 | CALORIES: 231 per serving

1⅓ cups raw Brazil nuts, soaked in water overnight
¼ cup lemon juice
¼ cup flaxseed oil
2 cloves garlic, peeled
1 teaspoon salt
¼ cup water
2 tablespoons chopped fresh parsley
2 tablespoons chopped fresh rosemary
1 tablespoon chopped fresh thyme
½ teaspoon ground black pepper
olive oil, for drizzling

Preheat the oven to 350°F and coat a rimmed baking sheet with cooking spray. Drain the water from the nuts and place in a food processor with the lemon juice, 3 tablespoons of the flaxseed oil, and the garlic, salt, and ¼ cup water. Blend until smooth and creamy. Line a 1-quart bowl with a clean kitchen towel or a piece of cheesecloth; spoon the mixture into the center of the towel. Bring the corners and sides of the towel together and twist around until it forms a grapefruit-size ball. Squeeze and extract excess liquid. Next, combine the parsley, rosemary, thyme, and pepper in a bowl. Unwrap the "cheese" ball and coat with the herbs. Place on the prepared baking sheet and bake for 30 minutes, or until the ball begins to crack. Remove from the oven, drizzle with olive oil, and serve warm with fresh vegetables, if desired.

Seeds

Simple Bowl of Buckwheat Groats

SERVES: 2 | CALORIES: 78 per serving

1 cup buckwheat

Rinse the groats three full times, draining the water quickly to preserve the groats' texture. Bring 2 cups of water to a boil, then add the buckwheat, cover with a lid, and turn the heat down. Cook for 15 to 20 minutes, until all the water is absorbed and the buckwheat is cooked Remove from the heat and let sit for another 10 minutes. It's especially yummy with dark leafy greens, as well as beans and legumes.

Bean and Buckwheat Soup

SERVES: 4 | CALORIES: 144 per serving

1 tablespoon olive oil
3 cloves garlic, minced (about 1 tablespoon)
¼ cup buckwheat groats
1 teaspoon chili powder
2 cups low-sodium vegetable broth
1½ cups cooked beans (any kind)
1 cup shredded carrots
2 cups water
¼ cup chopped watercress
2 tablespoons lemon juice
salt and pepper

Heat the oil in a saucepan over medium heat. Add the garlic, buckwheat, and chili powder, and sauté for 3 minutes. Stir in the broth, beans, carrots, and water, and season to taste with salt and pepper. Cover and bring to a boil. Reduce the heat to medium–low, and simmer for 20 minutes, or until the buckwheat groats are tender. Stir in the watercress and lemon juice.

Chia Seed Munchies

Refrigerate chia seeds to keep them fresh, and eat 1 to 2 tablespoons daily. You can also mix the seeds into your salads, juices, or smoothies.

Calories: 60 per tablespoon

Cha Cha Chia–Enriched Oatmeal

SERVES: 4 | CALORIES: 260 per serving

1 cup steel-cut oats

1 cup hemp milk

2 tablespoons chia seeds

¼ teaspoon ground cinnamon

pinch ground nutmeg

pinch black pepper

1 tablespoon shredded coconut

1 tablespoon chopped walnuts

Combine the oats, hemp milk, chia seeds, cinnamon, nutmeg, and black pepper in a glass jar with a lid. Tightly seal and refrigerate overnight. The next morning, stir and sprinkle with coconut and walnuts.

A WORD ABOUT FLAXSEED

Flaxseeds are high in calories, so pay special attention to portion size. You may want to add 1 or 2 tablespoons to your salads, soups, and steamed vegetables. Flaxseeds lose their powerhouse of nutrition when they're cooked, so it's best to opt for raw. You may want to add ground seeds to your cereal or smoothies and juices.

Calories: 55 per tablespoon

Flaxseed Salad Dressing

SERVES 6 | CALORIES: 50 per tablespoon

3 tablespoons lemon juice
1 large clove garlic
1 tablespoon chopped chives
3 tablespoons flaxseed oil
pinch cayenne pepper
½ teaspoon salt
black pepper

In a blender or food processor combine the lemon juice and garlic and blend until smooth. With the blender running, slowly add the oil in a fine stream and blend until slightly creamy. Add the chives, then season with salt and black pepper, to taste. Store leftovers in the refrigerator.

Hemp Seed Carrot Salad

SERVES: 2 | CALORIES: 278 per serving

2 medium carrots, peeled
¼ cup chopped onion
1 tablespoon shelled hemp seeds
2 teaspoons white wine vinegar
1 tablespoon hemp seed oil

Finely shred the carrots into a medium bowl. Stir in the onions and hemp seeds. In a small bowl, whisk the vinegar and hemp seed oil together. Add to the carrot mixture and toss to combine.

Hemp Seed Super Cereal

SERVES: 1 | CALORIES: 383

¼ cup raw sunflower seeds

2 tablespoons hemp seeds

2 tablespoons dried black currants

1 tablespoon shredded raw, unsweetened coconut

½ teaspoon ground cinnamon

⅛ teaspoon salt

1 teaspoon raw honey (optional; add 64 calories)

Mix all the ingredients together to combine.

Crunchy Sunflower Treat

SERVES: 1 | CALORIES: 340

1 quart water

¼ cup salt (optional)

½ cup sunflower seeds

Pour the water and salt, if using, into a saucepan over high heat. Rinse the sunflower seeds and add to the pan. Once the water boils, reduce the heat to a simmer and continue simmering for 1 full hour. Remove from the heat, drain the sunflower seeds, and spread them on a paper towel and allow to dry. Preheat the oven to 350°F. Spread the sunflower seeds on a rimmed baking sheet and bake for 25 to 30 minutes. Stir a few times. When the seeds are slightly brown and smelling heavenly, remove from the oven.

Sunflower Spread

CALORIES: 220 per tablespoon

2 cups sunflower seeds
½ cup tahini
¼ cup lemon juice
1 clove garlic, minced
¼ tablespoon minced onion (optional)
½ cup water

Toast the sunflower seeds in a frying pan over medium heat for 8 to 10 minutes, stirring continuously, until lightly browned. Transfer the hot seeds to a bowl and mix well with the tahini, stirring well to coat all the seeds. Spread the seeds out in a single layer and cool to room temperature. While cooling, combine the lemon juice and garlic in a small bowl. Set aside. Put the seeds in a food processor or hand–held blender along with the juice mixture, minced onion, and water; blend until the mixture is fairly fine. Cover and refrigerate if you're not using the spread within 15 minutes. If the spread firms up, stir in a tablespoon of water.

Spread on slices of 1 medium apple for an additional 72 calories.

Wheat Germ Cereal

SERVES: 2 | CALORIES: 104 per serving

¼ teaspoon salt
½ cup wheat germ

Place a double boiler on top of your stove. Remove the top half of the pot and fill the bottom half–way with water. Heat the water to boiling. Replace the top on the double boiler. Pour a pint of water into the upper part of the double boiler. Add the salt and bring the water to a boil. Sprinkle the wheat germ into the top of the double boiler slowly and leave on for 6 minutes. Stir the wheat germ continually while it cooks. After 6 minutes, place the lid on the double boiler and continue to cook the wheat germ cereal for an additional 30 minutes.

You can also add wheat germ to smoothies and soups.

Fruit

Baked Apple

SERVES: 1 | CALORIES: 100

1 medium Granny Smith apple
¼ teaspoon ground cinnamon
1 teaspoon black currants

Preheat the oven to 350°F. Wash the apple and scoop out the seeds and core while keeping the bottom intact. Combine the cinnamon and black currants in a cup. Fill the cored apple with the mixture. Bake in a shallow baking dish for 25 minutes.

Awesome Apple Sauce

SERVES: 2 | CALORIES: 80 per serving

2 apples peeled, cored, and chopped
½ cup water
¼ teaspoon ground cinnamon

In a saucepan, combine the apples, water, and cinnamon. Cover, and cook over medium heat for 15 to 20 minutes, or until the apples are soft. Allow to cool, then mash with a fork.

Low–Cal Guacamole

SERVES: 2 | CALORIES: 138 per serving

1½ tablespoons coarsely chopped red onion
1 tablespoon fresh lime juice
⅛ teaspoon salt
1 clove garlic
½ small jalapeño pepper
1 ripe avocado, peeled and pitted

Place the onion, lime juice, salt, garlic, and jalapeño in a food processor; pulse until finely chopped. Add the avocado and pulse until creamy.

Black Currant and Walnut Trail Mix

SERVES: 1 | CALORIES: 298

¼ cup walnuts
¼ cup dried black currants

Put ingredients in a jar and shake until mixed.

Berries Good

SERVES: 2 | CALORIES: about 100 per serving

½ pint strawberries, quartered
½ pint blueberries
½ pint fresh raspberries

Gently mix the berries together to combine.

Refreshing Coconut Milk

SERVES 4 | CALORIES: 60 calories per cup

Younger coconuts have soft flesh on the inside, which makes them easier to handle.

2 small young coconuts
pinch salt

Break open the coconuts with a heavy cleaver. Pour the liquid into the blender. Be careful to strain out any pieces of coconut shell or husk that may be in the liquid. Next scoop out the flesh with a spoon (this may take vigor) and add it to the blender. Blend on high for 1 minute and then strain the mixture through a cheesecloth or clean nylon stocking. Pour it back into the blender, add the salt, and blend again for 15 seconds. Transfer to an airtight jar and keep refrigerated. Can stay fresh for up to 5 days.

For a sweet accent, sprinkle shredded coconut on salads, sautéed vegetables, and fruit salads.
Calories: 40 per tablespoon

Hydrating Goji Berry Water

SERVES: 1 | CALORIES: 34 per cup

1 large handful goji berries
1 cup room-temperature water

Soak goji berries for at least 3 hours in water, stirring occasionally. Pour through a strainer to remove berries.

Crunchy Grape and Broccoli Salad

SERVES: 4 | CALORIES: 64 per serving

2 cups chopped raw broccoli
1 cup red grapes, halved
½ cup chopped onion
¼ cup sliced almonds
½ teaspoon lemon juice

Combine the broccoli, grapes, and onions in a bowl. Add sliced almonds. Mix well with the lemon juice.

Caramelized White Grapefruit

SERVES: 2 | CALORIES: 100 per serving

1 grapefruit
2 teaspoons agave nectar
2 pinches ground cinnamon (optional)

Wash the grapefruit and cut it in half. Cut around the outside of the grapefruit with a paring knife. Top each half with one teaspoon of agave. Sprinkle with cinnamon, if using. Broil for 3 minutes, or until grapefruit starts to caramelize. Eat warm.

Olé! Kiwi Salsa!

SERVES: 2 | CALORIES: 128 per serving

2 kiwis, peeled and diced
¼ sweet onion, diced
¼ jalapeno pepper, chopped
¼ teaspoon honey
⅛ teaspoon ground cumin
pinch cilantro
juice of ½ lemon
salt and pepper

Mix all the ingredients together in a bowl then cover and refrigerate for 30 minutes. Season with salt and pepper to taste.

Keep refrigerated until you're ready to eat. Add 72 calories if spread on a medium apple to serve.

Sweet Sliced Orange

SERVES: 2 | CALORIES: 197 per serving

2 oranges
1½ tablespoons honey
1 cinnamon stick
½ tablespoon water
1½ tablespoons sliced almonds, lightly toasted

Cut off peel and the pith (stringy white stuff) from the oranges. Slice the oranges into thin rounds using a serrated knife. Place the orange slices in a shallow bowl. Combine the honey, cinnamon stick, and water in a small saucepan and stir over low heat until the mixture comes to a simmer, about 2 minutes. Pour the syrup over the oranges while it's hot. Let cool. Sprinkle the almonds over the oranges. Serve cold or at room temperature. Store any extra portions in the refrigerator overnight. Keep covered.

Watermelon and Tomato Salad

SERVES: 2 | CALORIES: 188 per serving

2 medium ripe tomatoes, cut into ¾-inch chunks
½ cup chopped seedless watermelon, in ¾-inch cubes
½ avocado, peeled, pitted, and cut into ¾-inch cubes
½ tablespoon chopped chives and/or cilantro
1½ tablespoons extra-virgin olive oil
1½ tablespoons aged balsamic vinegar
salt and pepper

Combine the tomatoes, watermelon, avocado, and herbs in a bowl. In a small bowl, whisk together the olive oil, balsamic vinegar, and salt and pepper to taste. Pour the dressing over the tomato mixture and toss to coat.

Vegetables

Three Bean Salad

SERVES: 3 | CALORIES: 137 per serving

½ cup canned cannellini beans
½ cup canned kidney beans
½ cup canned chickpeas
¼ red onion, finely chopped
½ cup fresh finely chopped watercress
¼ cup lemon juice
1 teaspoon salt
¼ teaspoon pepper

In a large bowl, mix the beans, onion, and watercress. In a separate small bowl, whisk together the lemon juice, salt, pepper, and add the dressing to the beans. Toss to coat. Refrigerate, covered, for several hours to allow the beans to soak up the flavor of the dressing.

Nutty Steamed Broccoli

SERVES: 4 | CALORIES: 165 per servings

1 bunch broccoli
1 tablespoon flaxseed oil
juice of ½ squeezed lemon
¼ cup sliced raw almonds

Break the broccoli into bite-size florets. Quarter the stems lengthwise. Bring ¾ to 1 inch of water to a boil in a saucepan with a steamer basket. Add the broccoli to the steamer and cover; reduce the heat to medium and let cook for 5 to 6 minutes, until you can pierce with a fork. Don't overcook! Remove from the heat, place in a dish, and stir in the lemon juice and almonds.

Non–Dairy Coleslaw with Black Currants

SERVES: 4 | CALORIES: 109 per serving

2 finely shredded cups cabbage
1 apple, peeled and chopped
1 small carrot, chopped
½ small red onion, chopped
¼ cup black currants
2 tablespoons flaxseed oil
½ teaspoon chopped parsley
salt and pepper

Toss the shredded cabbage, apple, carrot, red onion, and black currants in a large bowl. Drizzle sparingly with flaxseed oil. Add the parsley and toss to combine. Season with salt and pepper to taste.

Carrot Walnut Salad with Goji Berries

SERVES: 7 | CALORIES: 115 per serving

½ cup goji berries
½ cup raw walnuts, divided
2 tablespoons lemon juice
1 pound carrots
salt

Place the goji berries in a bowl and cover with hot water. Soak until plump, then drain. Place 2 tablespoons berries, ¼ cup of the walnuts, and the lemon juice in a blender on high speed until liquefied. Trim and cut the carrots so they can fit into a large feeding tube or food processor (with the disc on shred), then shred carrots in several batches. Put in a big bowl, stir in the walnut mixture, and salt and pepper to taste. Stir in the remaining goji berries and walnuts. Refrigerate for at least 2 hours. Stir again before serving. Store in the refrigerator in an airtight container.

Roasted Garlic

CALORIES: 110

1 garlic bulb
1 teaspoon olive oil

Preheat the oven to 400°F. Peel away the outer layers of
the garlic bulb skin, but leave the skins on the individual
cloves. Cut off ½ inch from the top of the bulb to expose the
individual cloves. Place the garlic head in a baking pan. Drizzle
a couple teaspoons of olive oil over the head then rub gently
with finger tips to be sure it's completely coated. Cover with
aluminum foil. Bake for 30 to 35 minutes, or until the cloves
feel soft when pressed. Allow to cool before eating.

A NOTE ABOUT LEAFY GREENS

All dark green leafy vegetables can be considered superfoods,
and steaming is an excellent way to get the most nutritional
value with the least number of calories. Follow these
directions to cook succulent greens:

Cut or trim your greens into smaller pieces first. A steaming
basket is a cheap way to steam food. Fill a pot with 2 ounces
of water, place a steaming basket with cut greens on top, and
cover with a lid. Once the water boils, steam until tender for
about 3 minutes, depending on the green. While the greens
cook, fill a bowl with ice water. Immediately after steaming,
plunge the greens into the ice bath to stop the cooking
process so your greens remain a little crunchy and retain
their color.

Calories: About 125 per 1–cup serving

Roasted Radishes

SERVES: 4 | CALORIES: 37 per serving

1 bunch small to medium radishes (about 12)
1 tablespoon olive oil
1 teaspoon dried thyme
salt and pepper
juice of ½ lemon

Preheat the oven to 450°F. Place the radishes on a baking sheet and toss with the olive oil, thyme, salt, and pepper. Roast until tender yet still firm in the center, about 20 minutes. Squeeze with a little lemon juice and serve.

Roasted Sweet Potato

SERVES: 1 | CALORIES: 185

1 small sweet potato
½ teaspoon olive oil
1 teaspoon minced fresh rosemary
salt to taste

Preheat the oven to 450°F. Cut the sweet potato lengthwise into slim wedges. In a large bowl, combine the sweet potato, olive oil, and rosemary. Season with salt to taste. Arrange the sweet potato wedges in a single layer on a baking sheet. Bake for 30 minutes, turning after 15 minutes. Serve immediately.

Juicy Sliced Tomato and Watercress

SERVES: 2 | CALORIES: 66 per serving

2 ripe tomatoes (preferably heirloom)
½ tablespoon olive oil
½ cup chopped watercress
salt and pepper

Thinly the slice tomatoes, drizzle with olive oil, and sprinkle with chopped watercress. Season with salt and pepper to taste.

Watercress Pesto

SERVES 2 | CALORIES: 103 per serving (without the apple or radish)

1 clove garlic
¼ cup walnuts
1 cup watercress

Place the garlic, walnuts, and watercress in a food processor or blender. Pulse until a finely chopped paste has formed. Serve on apple or radish slices.

Feel like a dessert? *Treat yourself to an ounce of dark chocolate!*

Calories: 155

6

Beyond Calorie Counting

There are two ways to live: you can live as if nothing is a
miracle; you can live as if everything is a miracle.
~Albert Einstein

Confession: The first time I tried a two–day cleanse more than
a decade ago, I was sure I would never get through it. And I
didn't. Three hours into the regimen I was sneaking handfuls of
chips and later in the day stopping by the store for a package
of Gummy Bears (my faves). But instead of feeling better, I felt
worse about myself. Not only had I blown the diet but I was
still a victim to my cravings. I felt weak. In those bad ol' days, I
had a crummy attitude. I wanted to achieve results without any
effort. I wanted a *miracle*.

It took me several tries before I fully mastered cleansing, and
when I finally did, it was because I surrendered to deep inner
and outer work. Counting calories is one thing, but embracing
a new way of dealing with life is another. I learned to welcome

a physically and emotionally nontoxic and reduced-stress life. I did a clean sweep of my environment and introduced practices to help reduce conflicts within myself.

This much I know: If you make the Two-Day Superfood Cleanse a regular part of your life, you'll feel more alive. You might even sense a state of utter exhilaration. Your life *will* change. Stress, random thoughts, impatience, unhappiness, body fatigue, stiffness, and that bloated feeling will drain away. You may, for the first time in your life, get glimpses of being truly at peace with a clear, uncritical mind and an open, loving heart. You'll also look great. Miracles do happen. But you have to be open and prepared to receive them ... and you need to stay the course.

This final chapter offers you dozens of ways to support your regular Two-Day Superfood Cleanse. You might feel resistance to certain practices, but keep in mind that they're probably the very ones you most need to incorporate into your life. Give them a try.

Your Outer World

Eliminating unhealthy, processed, and pesticide-filled foods is only part of the issue when it comes to cleansing. The other part is paying attention to toxins in your environment that may be interfering with your breathing, hormones, cellular balance, biochemistry, and stress levels and in the process causing headaches, stomach upset, skin outbreaks, moodiness, weight gain, and a host of other ailments.

What to do? Start with a clean sweep of your house by removing everything from cleaning products to cosmetics that may be causing you harm. Here are the top offenders:

NIX PLASTIC CONTAINERS: Stay away from cling wrap, cooking oil in plastic bottles, Styrofoam containers, and hard plastic drinking bottles, cups, and dishes. They all contain polyvinyl chloride (V or PVC) or polystyrene. Instead, store your leftovers in glass or ceramic containers. When you're buying food to-go, refuse Styrofoam and plastic. Order from restaurants that put your food in paper and cardboard. Of course you already know this, but never, *ever* microwave food in plastic. FYI: I'm not a big fan of microwaving, anyway.

OPT FOR NATURAL FIBER LINENS: Conventional mattresses usually contain petrochemicals, flame retardants, dyes, PVC, phthalates, and more. The same may go for towels and other linens. Invest in organic sheets and a natural fabric mattress labeled "organic." They're more expensive but you'll sleep better knowing you're not being poisoned.

CONSIDER REDECORATING: Does your home need a new paint job? Good! If you can't afford to do the whole house, at least consider using nontoxic paints in your bedroom (where you spend a lot of time) and bathroom (where steam can allow toxic fumes to enter through your skin and lungs). The best option is VOC-free paints, which use water instead of petroleum-based solvents and contain no heavy metals or formaldehyde. These paints are readily available at most home improvement stores.

GET INTO GREENERY: According to the Environmental Protection Agency (EPA), our indoor air can be two to five times more polluted than the outdoor air we breathe. House plants help to rid the air of pollutants and toxins, counteracting out-gassing and contributing to balanced internal humidity. If you don't have a green thumb, choose plants that require nothing more than a once-a-week watering, such as aloe, jade, or peace lily.

BACK OFF FROM BLEACH: The EPA also found that chlorine byproducts (known as dioxins) are 300,000 more times as carcinogenic as the scary chemical pesticide DDT. It's not only the bleach that you pour into your laundry that's worrisome, you'll need to cut out bleached paper products like paper towels, toilet paper, and bleached coffee filters. Substitute with chlorine-free (or PCF) paper products.

SAY *TA-TA* TO TEFLON: Yeah, nonstick pots are a breeze to clean but you may be getting poisoned in the process. Studies have shown that this kind of cookware may damage your thyroid and liver, as well as weaken your immune system. Replace all nonstick cookware with iron, porcelain-coated, stainless steel, or glass pots and pans. Remember—a little elbow grease never hurt anyone; it helps burn calories.

TAKE CARE WITH DRY CLEANING: If you've ever taken your clothes to a professional dry cleaner, the likelihood that they were cleaned with dangerous chemicals is high. According to Occidental College's Pollution Prevention Center, 85 percent of the more than 35,000 dry cleaners in the United States use perchloroethylene (or perc, for short) as a solvent in the dry cleaning process. The good news is that there are nontoxic cleaning alternatives that are just as effective as dry cleaning with perc. Only go to dry cleaners that are certified "green." Or bite the bullet and hand wash your garments with all-natural soap products.

Three Simple and Inexpensive Natural Homemade Cleaning Products

1 **VINEGAR AND WATER:** Vinegar has disinfecting properties and can be used as a multipurpose cleaner in the bathroom and kitchen to clean floors, mirrors, and windows. It's even an effective natural stain remover. Mix white vinegar with water in a 1:1 ratio in a spray bottle. Warning: Don't use on porous surfaces like granite or marble.

2 **BAKING SODA:** Sprinkle in the toilet, sink, and shower as an abrasive cleaner. If you have a carpet, sprinkle before vacuuming as an added disinfectant and deodorizer.

3   **HYDROGEN PEROXIDE AND WATER:** While a mixture of half water, half hydrogen peroxide is perfect for using in places that you really want to make sure are completely disinfected (like the kitchen countertop after working with raw meat, or the bathroom pretty much anytime). It's especially helpful after someone in your family is sick. It's important to keep the hydrogen peroxide mixture in its dark brown bottle because the fluid breaks down when exposed to light.

While You're at It, Clean Up Your Medicine Cabinet and Throw Away:

EXPIRED MEDICINES: They lose their effectiveness and in some instances can become dangerous. Check expiration dates thoroughly.

NEARLY EMPTY BOTTLES: They not only create clutter but may not even have enough medicine left for a full dose.

IMPROPERLY STORED ITEMS: They can partially evaporate, leaving them more concentrated and dangerous. Get rid of items that were not sealed or stored properly.

OLD PRESCRIPTIONS OR PARTIALLY USED PRESCRIPTIONS: Check with your physician if you have questions about saving prescriptions.

Not-So Gorgeous Cosmetics

Every morning after the average American woman wakes up, she smears, cakes, sprays, dots, and powders around 12 different health and beauty products on her face and body before leaving home. But plenty of these products contain harsh chemicals that have been linked to cancer and organ failure, even birth defects. Why doesn't the FDA do something about it? Well, cosmetics aren't subject to the same oversight as food and pharmaceuticals. It's up to the cosmetic manufacturer to decide whether a product is safe, and you can imagine how much credibility that gives a seal of approval.

But the Environmental Working Group has come to our rescue and outed cosmetics containing chemicals with known, or suspected, health risks. The nonprofit group considers each of the following to be "high hazard," based on information provided by the U.S. government and scientific studies.

CERTAIN SUNSCREENS: The sunscreen ingredient known as octinoxate may help filter UV rays, but it's also been linked to thyroid and brain signal problems in lab animals. The "natural" label stamped on a cosmetic sunscreen puts it in the fastest-growing sales category, but it's no guarantee the ingredients are safe.

FOUNDATION FAILURES: Oxybenzone can be a double-edged ingredient. Frequently included as an ingredient in facial foundations for protection against UV rays, it causes irritation or may trigger allergic reactions to light. The chemical may also be absorbed by skin. According to the U.S. Centers for Disease Control & Prevention, 97 percent of Americans have built up some amount of this chemical in their bodies.

SHINE-REDUCING POWDER: Women who use this kind of product to get rid of shine on top of their concealer may be getting a double dose of retinyl palmitate, which has been linked to cancer in lab animals. For coloring, some powders use "lake" dyes, which contain metals such as aluminum, calcium, and barium, known neurotoxins that are still allowed by the FDA for cosmetic uses in limited amounts.

BAD MINERAL BLUSH: Rose quartz and silica are included in some mineral blushes in order to offer a powdery and glittery finish. Unfortunately, there's nothing shiny about these ingredients. They're both considered possible human carcinogens and have proven toxic to immune and respiratory systems over prolonged exposure.

MALEVOLENT MASCARA: This beauty product may seem an odd place to find fragrance ingredients, but manufacturers often include it in mascara to disguise unpleasant chemical odors. Certain fragrances can set off headaches, wheezing, and asthma in a concoction of compounds. Some mascaras also include retinyl palmitate and parabens, which are used as preservatives and can mimic estrogen and interfere with the endocrine system.

HEALTH-DIMMING EYE SHADOW: Retinyl palmitate, parabens, and "lake" dyes are also included in certain eye shadows. Many also contain ingredients that increase absorption into the skin, multiplying the potential health risk.

LOSER LIPSTICKS: Far from perking up your lips, some rejuvenators contain retinyl palmitate, oxybenzone, and undisclosed fragrance chemicals. Certain brands of lipstick also still contain lead, which can be ingested and accumulate in the body, potentially causing learning and behavioral disorders.

FRAGRANCE FAILURES: Even though plenty of perfumes and colognes really do contain trace amounts of natural essences, they typically also possess over a dozen potentially hazardous synthetic chemicals; many are derived from petroleum.

Your Inner Life

Following the Breath
Breathing in, I calm my body.
Breathing out, I smile.
Dwelling in the present moment,
I know this is a wonderful moment!

> *~ Thich Nhat Hanh,*
> *Vietnamese Zen*
> *Buddhist Monk*

Deep Breathing

Do you think there's a big spiritual secret to deep breathing? There isn't. This is all you have to do:

Consciously exhale a long and thin breath through your nose. Feel it on your upper lip. Then inhale slowly through the center of both nostrils. Pause. Try it again. If your exhale was shallow, try exhaling through your mouth with the sound "ahh" to explore the length of your exhale. Then do it several times through your nose again.

This kind of very simple mindful or conscious breath puts you in the moment. It demands your attention to be in the now. Eastern yogic philosophy claims we are allotted a certain number of breaths per lifetime. In the West, we've proven that stress is related to diseases and that long, deep breathing helps reduce stress. Think about it: Breathing is the first thing we do when we are born and the last thing we do when we die.

When you are new to the practice, you may choose to close your eyes so your attention is on the breath and not on outside activities and scenery. However, eventually you actually want to do this practice with your eyes open, aware of your environment. This way, you learn to connect to your breath as you are moving regularly from moment to moment, engaged in the world around you. With eyes open, you can practice observing your breath throughout your day.

Benefits of deep breathing:
- Strengthens respiratory and immune systems
- Reduces stress
- Revitalizes the body
- Refreshes the brain
- Promotes healing on emotional and physical levels
- Puts consciousness in the present
- Trains the brain to let go during exhales

Make It with Meditation

You should sit in meditation for 20 minutes a day, unless you're too busy; then you should sit for an hour.

~ Zen saying

When it comes to making meditation a part of your daily routine, metaphorically speaking, it's a no-brainer. Studies show meditation does everything from taming the runaway "monkey mind," increasing creativity, and pumping up energy and vitality to reducing muscle pain, lowering stress, boosting organizational skills, and offering mental and physical flexibility.

The ability to quiet one's mind and retreat to a thought-free state of calmness opens the connection to higher intelligence and greatly enhances problem-solving abilities. A study at Massachusetts General Hospital found that the cerebral cortex (the part of the brain that deals with focusing on processing sensory input) is more active in meditators.

The science confirming meditation's benefits is far-reaching. Here's just a snapshot taken from hundreds of available studies:

- Of hypertensive meditation patients who meditated, 80 percent lowered their blood pressure and decreased medications, while 16 percent were able to discontinue using their medication all together, according to a Harvard Medical School study.

- Researchers at Northwestern Memorial Hospital in Chicago found that people with insomnia who meditated for 15 to 20 minutes twice daily for two months *all* reported improved sleep; in fact, the majority of them were able to reduce or eliminate sleeping medication.

- Folks who suffered from chronic pain, including that from injury, surgery, arthritis, and fibromyalgia, reduced their physician visits by 42 percent, and open–heart surgery patients had fewer postoperative complications due to a regular practice of meditation, according to studies conducted at the University of Pittsburgh Medical Center.

- Researchers at Cedars–Sinai Medical Center in Los Angeles showed that patients were able to lower their blood sugar and insulin by practicing meditation.

- The *Journal of Obstetrics and Gynecology* reports that women with severe PMS who meditate daily have a 57 percent reduction in physical and psychological symptoms.

If findings like these don't give you enough reason to consider placing your butt on a cushion, how about meditation's ability to add years to your life? The *International Journal of Neuroscience* reports that meditators who have been practicing for at least five years are physiologically twelve years younger than their non–meditating counterparts. The reasons? Studies show meditators lower their levels of cholesterol, blood sugar, inflammation, and the stress hormone cortisol – all of which are known agers.

What's more, studies done by Yale, Harvard, and Massachusetts General Hospital have shown that meditation increases gray matter in the brain and slows down certain kinds of brain deterioration. The Harvard experiment included 20 individuals with intensive Buddhist "insight meditation" training and 15 who did not meditate. The brain scan revealed that those who meditated have an increased thickness of gray matter in parts of the brain that are responsible for attention. There are dozens more studies proving meditation decreases depression, anxiety, and moodiness and boosts self–esteem, concentration, and relaxation. The practice simply makes people happier. It reminds us of our purpose in life: to experience *joy* in the here and now.

Meditation also produces a state of relaxation, relief from stress, and helps to eliminate feelings of anxiety and anger. Using a moving MRI, researchers at the University of Wisconsin looked at the brains of meditators and discovered their amygdala (the part of the brain responsible for the fight–or–flight impulse) switches off and the prefrontal cortex, the area of the brain responsible for feelings of peace, compassion, and happiness, lights up. Meditation is the perfect antidote, especially for stress junkies, particularly in our culture. Consider it a tool. When you make a commitment to a Superfood Cleanse where the aim is for self–improvement, mediation takes you one step further. It helps make your life even better.

How to Meditate

Although meditation has profound effects on our well-being and our openness to cleanse, it doesn't have to be a complicated process. Advanced meditators may prefer to sit on a cushion in a lotus or half–lotus position and focus on their breathing or on a particular chakra (one of the seven centers of spiritual energy in the human body, according to yogic philosophy), but beginners can follow these basic steps:

- Sit in a quiet, comfortable place in a straight–back chair or on a floor cushion. Relax your muscles; do not lie down.
- Select a syllable, phrase, or word, such as "one," "peace," "love," or "om" to focus on.
- Close your eyes and follow the rhythm of your breath.
- Repeat your chosen word as you breathe in and out. If your mind wanders, don't quit. Just let your thoughts go and refocus by repeating your chosen word.
- Continue for 10 to 20 minutes.

When you finish, sit quietly for a minute or two – one first with eyes closed, then with eyes open – and enjoy life.

Helpful Hints for Beginners

START SMALL: Try meditating for only five minutes to start. It's not really the length of time that's important but the regularity of the practice.

SET A FIXED TIME: If you keep changing the time, there's a good chance that you're going to forget to meditate some days, and then the practice dies out. So pick a specific time. Morning is often best, but choose what works best for you.

FIND A SPECIAL SPOT: Ideally you want a place that is "reserved" for this practice, a "retreat" space. It needn't be a temple in your home. It can be a small pillow in the corner of a room, a chair in your bedroom or on your bed. Wherever you choose, it should be quiet, clean, and dedicated to the practice.

KEEP A TIMER HANDY: You should use a timer so you never have to guess how long you've meditated. You can use your phone timer (while in airplane mode) or a meditation app, which will give you a nice gong at the beginning and end of your set time.

Mindful Eating

Be honest. How often do you really revel in the taste of the food you're eating? Maybe the first few bites, but then if you're like most us, you slip into a near unconscious state. Now imagine being fully present for every mouthful. You're tasting every flavor and feeling every sensation of texture. Try putting a mindful eating exercise into practice during your 600–calorie Superfood Cleanse days and make the most of every bite. Here's how:

- Sit down at a table, preferably alone, and free from any external distractions. Don't worry too much if there are sounds that are out of your control; you can build these into the exercise. Before you even pick up the food to eat, take a couple of deep breaths – in through the nose and out through the mouth–to allow the body and mind to settle.

- Take a moment to think about the food. Where has it come from? What country? Try to imagine the different ingredients in their natural growing environment.

- Take note: Are you feeling any impatience? Do you want to get on with it and just eat? Perhaps you're thinking of all the things you need to do. Whatever the reaction, it's most likely just conditioned behavior–a habit–but one that you may find surprisingly strong. Regardless of the feeling, take at least a minute to reflect on it.

- Allow time to appreciate the food on your plate. Remember there are many people in the world who are hungry. A deep sense of gratitude is at the heart of any mindfulness practice.

- If it's a food you're going to eat with your hands, notice the texture as you pick it up, the temperature, and perhaps the colors. If you're eating from a plate with a knife and fork, notice instead the texture and temperature of the cutlery as you move it toward the food. You might find it more effective to hold your fork or spoon in your nondominant hand: This will prevent you from going too quickly.

- How does the food smell? What does it look like up close? As you put it in your mouth, what is the taste, the texture, the temperature? You don't need to "do" anything. Simply observe the experience of your senses.

- Take the time to chew your food completely. Not only is this a healthier way of eating, but it will allow you the time to taste and appreciate all the different flavors.

- When you've finished eating the food on your plate, before standing up and moving onto the next thing you have planned, try staying seated for a moment or two. This is an opportunity for you to take that sense of being present to the next part of your day.

Journal Writing

During the course of your cleanse days it's possible you'll have numerous creative thoughts or memories swirling around. You may envision a new project, remember an event in your childhood, appreciate a sunset, or feel sudden tenderness toward an old friend. Writing down your thoughts and keeping a journal is a wonderful way to record and embrace your life during these deepening days.

You can use your journal as a private way to explore your thoughts and delve into your psyche, or you may choose to share it with others. Many people write as a way to share their personal history. But the most important part of writing in your journal is that it offers you a chance to be utterly truthful.

Keeping an honest journal not only has emotional benefits but physical ones as well. One study found that subjects who had composed an accurate account of their personal tribulations made two–thirds fewer trips to the doctor than the group that wrote fictional or impersonal accounts. Writing openly, researchers suggest, may help us develop a sense of control over our emotions, and this in turn may contribute to good health.

How to Keep a Journal

- You can write down your thoughts, your feelings, your dreams, and your observations. It's important to try to write every day of your cleanse. Remember, these writings are not for publication (unless you choose them to be), so you need not fret about the sentence structure or, more importantly, the subject matter. You will be less inhibited if your writings are just between you and a notebook.

- Writing is therapeutic. It gives you the opportunity to take stock of yourself, think about how you feel, and express your opinions. Think of it as a forum for self–analysis. Try not to dwell on negative emotions. If those are the only ones you explore, try learning something about what you are feeling and imagine ways to change your emotions. Write down these thoughts, too.

- Affirmations, biblical proverbs, poems, excerpts from stories, even song lyrics with special significance can be recorded in your journal. If you're a visual person, you may decide to draw or cut out images and paste them in your notebook; you can use these for inspiration.

- In any case, keep a journal for *you* and use it as a safe place to go during quiet times. Know that it is your private possession. There is a reason why many journals are designed with locks and keys. But it doesn't matter whether you buy a nice bound notebook–the aim is to just let your words flow. Keeping a journal is a personal journey.

Rise Early

I'm with Ben Franklin who, as most of us know, said, "Early to bed and early to rise makes a man healthy, wealthy, and wise." Rising at the crack of dawn has never been an issue for me. I can't wait to watch the sunrise as color sweeps across the sky, click on my computer and read last night's mail and today's news, and then settle on my cushion to meditate.

There are also scientifically based health reasons for waking early. Morning is when our blood sugar levels are the lowest. You've gone all night without food and your brain is off-kilter. Low blood sugar really affects your mood (adversely). Getting up three hours early allows you to preempt the blood sugar low and prematurely head it off at the pass by eating an early breakfast. Also, levels of the stress hormone cortisol are naturally highest in the early morning and when many people wake up. Waking up before cortisol levels peak allows you to save yourself from feeling stressed out and eating out of anxiety. Here are more morning perks:

- Gratitude will spring forth: Light on the horizon may inspire you to greet your day with gratitude, which studies show makes us generally happier and more positive people. This is what the Dali Lama says each morning:

  "Today I am fortunate to have woken up, I am alive, I have a precious human life, I am not going to waste it. I am going to use all my energies to develop myself, to expand my heart out to others, to achieve enlightenment for the benefit of all beings, I am going to have kind thoughts towards others, I am not going to get angry or think badly about others, I am going to benefit others as much as I can."

- You needn't bolt out of bed because you're rushing to get going and you're already late. Now you have time to stretch in bed, think about the day ahead, and then rise and get a real jump on your chores.

- You can enjoy the peace and quiet: little traffic outdoors, no television or radio blasting, and if you have kids or other family members in the house, they're still tucked in bed, which means no requests. This is time just for you.

- Time for breakfast juicing: If you get up before the day breaks, you can enjoy this meal's namesake. Don't skip it. Luxuriate in the first taste of the day. If it's only hot water and lemon you're enjoying, sip slowly.

- You can't beat morning exercise. Of course, there are other times to exercise besides the early morning. But now you don't have the hassles of the day behind you along with a million excuses. Research shows those who exercise in the morning are more likely to stick to a set routine.

- You can get stuff done. Studies conclude we're most productive in the midmornings. So you can line up your tasks upon awakening and be prepared when the jolt of can–do energy is peaking. Or use this time to tap into your creative side and keep a morning journal. You can also record your dreams.

Four Yoga Poses to Bump Up Your Metabolism

CHILD'S POSE: Begin by sitting on your heels with knees bent. To soften any strain on your knees place a yoga block or folded blanket between your feet. Using your eyes to guide you, revolve your body to the right, looking over your shoulder. Hold and breathe for a count of ten, return to the center, and revolve to the left in the same manner. Return to center.

Extend your hands and arms forward into pose of the child. Try to place your buttocks on your heels. If this is too difficult, open your knees wider and keep your feet together as you extend.

CAT/COW BREATHING: Get on all fours, making sure your hands are directly beneath your shoulders and your knees are right under your hips. Continue to breathe normally without forcing or "trying" to breathe. On the inhale, round up into Cat Stretch by tilting your pelvis upward and tucking your chin toward your chest. Round your back, keeping your arms straight and your hips aligned over your knees. On the exhale, tilt your pelvis downward while gently arching the back and looking upward to where the wall meets the ceiling.

Move between Cat and Cow stretch four to five times before stretching back into extended child's pose, finally rolling up to sit back on your heels. Repeat the entire sequence four to five times.

KNEE HUGGING: Lay on your back, legs extended out, and bring your right knee in toward your chest. Interlace your fingers around the knee. Your elbows are lifted up and out to the side to keep the lungs open. Without forcing the knee, round up and gaze down the length of the extended leg. Hold for the count of five, then roll down.

Lower the right leg and repeat with the left leg. Bring both knees into your chest, and then extend away to arm's length. Repeat in and away several times. This is a great massage for the lower digestive system, as well as, your lower back. Repeat the entire sequence four to five times then extend the legs out.

TWIST: Laying on your back, bring both knees in toward your chest and wrap your arms around your knees as much as possible. Hold for the count of ten, breathing naturally. Release your knees, and while keeping them bent, move them out and over your hips. Extend your arms out to the side and ground your shoulders and palms of your hands to the floor. Slowly lower your feet and knees over to the right, keeping your shoulders and palms grounded. Plant your gaze toward the ceiling.

You can make the rotations with knees bent and feet off the floor; an easier way is to keep the feet flat and together on the floor and lower from one side to the other. Return to the center and lower your bent legs over to the left. Move your legs from right to left, inhaling to lift and exhaling to lower for four to five times. On the final rotation stay and hold on the right side for a count of ten. Then lift up and over to the left holding for ten counts.

Come back to the center, extend your legs, and rest before repeating the sequence.

Why You Should Be Walking

Going the distance on your feet can give you a huge health boost. For optimum results, it's recommended you try two miles at a brisk pace of three to four miles per hour nearly every day—or the so-called "Magic 10,000 Steps." Here's what you'll get out of it:

HELP THE HEART: University of South Carolina researchers followed 46,000 men and 15,000 women over the course of 18 years. They found those with increased fitness levels associated with regular brisk walking had a 40 percent lower risk of heart disease or stroke than those with the lowest fitness level.

KEEP YOU SLIM: According to research by Dr. James O. Hill of the Center for Human Nutrition at the University of Colorado Health Sciences Center, if you add just 2,000 steps a day to your regular activities, you may never gain another pound. But remember: Don't increase calories.

REDUCE CANCER RISK: Numerous studies report that walking and exercise reduce your risk of breast and colon cancer. In fact, walking is also good for those who are undergoing cancer treatment because it improves chances of recovery and survival.

CUT DOWN DIABETES: A study by the Graduate School of Public Health at the University of Pittsburgh discovered that walking for 30 minutes a day cut diabetes risks for overweight as well as non-overweight men and women. Walking also helps maintain blood sugar balance for those with diabetes.

RELIEVE STRESS: Walking leads to the release of the body's natural feel-good endorphins. A study published in the *Annals of Behavioral Medicine* showed that university students who walked regularly had lower stress levels than couch potatoes or even those who exercised strenuously.

ENHANCE YOUR SEX LIFE: In a study of women between 45 and 55 years old, those who exercised, which included brisk walking, reported not only greater sexual desire but better sexual satisfaction.

Dance! Dance! Dance!

Ballroom, jazz, tap, hip-hop, salsa, swing, or disco, even chair dancing–whatever your fancy–kicking up your heels (or pointing your toes) offers a fun way to stay fit and healthy. Here's what moving to the beat can do for you:

KEEP YOU SLIM: On average, a 150-pound adult can burn about 150 calories doing 30 minutes of moderate social dancing.

FIT YOUR PARTICULAR NEEDS: Unlike many other kinds of exercise, you can easily adjust the level of exertion just by putting in more enthusiasm or less. Although some dance forms are more rigorous than others–for instance, jazz as opposed to the waltz–all beginners' classes should start you out gradually.

WIDEN YOUR SOCIAL CIRCLE: When you join a dance club or class you'll have lots of opportunities to meet new people. Countless studies show the importance of socializing. Remember, you don't need to bring a partner–you'll find one there.

INCREASE HAPPINESS: Dancing is fun! And the more heart, soul, and sweat you put into it, the more the feel-good brain chemical, endorphins, will be released.

Try Reflexology

This type of foot massage was first developed in ancient China and is based on the same philosophy used in acupuncture. It works with the body's energy channels. Every part of the foot corresponds to a particular area of the body. The reflexologist stimulates the meridians of the feet through touch and massage, promoting healing and relaxation. Here's what a treatment from a licensed reflexologist can do for you:

RELAXATION: To reduce anxiety and calm the body down, the reflexologist walks the finger or thumb over different areas of your feet in a set sequence, massaging and kneading your foot using her whole hand. The experience should feel gentle, yet firm.

REDUCE PAIN: Several studies funded by the National Cancer Institute and the National Institutes of Health indicate that reflexology may reduce pain and enhance relaxation and sleep. Pressing on particular points on the feet can sometimes relieve headaches, back pain, arthritis, and other chronic pain conditions.

INCREASE CIRCULATION: The act of applying pressure to the feet stimulates blood flow to the area. Increased blood flow brings not only blood, but the oxygen and nutrients it transports to all areas of the body, promoting healing and well-being.

AID DIGESTION: There are specific points in the feet that correspond to the digestive organs. Placing pressure on these points helps to relieve digestive disorders.

REMOVE TOXINS: It's so effective at eliminating toxins in the body that most people feel a need to urinate after a session and are nearly always thirsty.

INDUCE SLEEP: For a more restful sleep, practitioners apply pressure to both big toes. The point on the outside of your big toe, just below the tip, corresponds with the pineal gland, which regulates the sleep hormone melatonin. Rubbing the rest of the big toe releases soothing endorphins, helping you relax. Try this one yourself.

The Health Benefits of a Cold Shower

A cold shower? Am I joking? Well, not exactly. There are real wellness benefits to ending your warm and cozy shower with a spray of cool, refreshing water, especially during your cleansing days. Here's what you'll gain:

INCREASED CIRCULATION: Although warm water makes the blood rush to your skin, cool water brings blood rushing to your organs. Ideally, you'll switch back and forth numerous times but just ending the shower with cold water helps with circulation. This boost can even help to reduce the appearance of varicose veins.

GLOWING SKIN: Begin with warm water, which will open your pores and make them receptive to cleaning. Then close your pores when you're done by rinsing with cool water. Another benefit is that cool water makes your blood vessels constrict, which reduces swelling and the appearance of dark circles under your eyes (where skin is at its thinnest).

SHINY HAIR: Simply, cold water makes your hair look healthier and shinier. That's why there's a cool air button on your hair dryer. Cold water works by closing the hair cuticle, which makes the hair stronger and prevents dirt from easily accumulating within your scalp.

MOOD BUMP: There are plenty of mental benefits to ending your shower with chilly water. The ancient samurai warriors used to pour buckets of cold river water on their heads every morning in a Shinto practice called *Misogi*. They believed it cleansed the spirit and helped start the day fresh, opening the heart and mind to new adventures. It can't be denied; cold water is energizing and invigorating. Give it a whirl. Guaranteed you'll feel the lift.

The key is not to torture yourself. Start gradually, making it a little colder and staying under the chilly spray a little longer each time you shower.

Listen to Music

It turns out you can't beat the sounds of music when it comes to supporting well-being. Several studies have shown it can lower anxiety, help sleep, increase brain power, decrease appetite, and encourage us to exercise.

REDUCE STRESS: It's no secret that stress triggers a host of illnesses. Research has shown that tuning into music can help reduce stress and anxiety while releasing feel-good hormones. According to a Japanese study, levels of stress hormones (ACTH and cortisol) were measured in surgical patients just before anesthesia was administered. Patients who listened to soothing music immediately before showed a drop in stress hormones by more than 50 percent. The opposite happened to those who did not listen to music; their hormone levels showed a rise of more than 50 percent.

HEIGHTEN BRAIN FUNCTION: Leigh Rigby and George Caldwell, cognitive psychologists at Glasgow Caledonian University, monitored the brain activity of a group of 16 volunteers who were asked to perform a simple memory test while listening to rock and classical music. They were asked to do the same while listening to the sound of static and again in silence. Brain scans revealed that subjects required far less brainpower to complete the test successfully when music was playing than when there was only static or silence.

UP EXERCISE EFFICIENCY: Syncing beats per minute while moving increases the effects of exercise. In a recent study, subjects who cycled in time to music found that they required 7 percent less oxygen to do the same work when compared to music playing in the background. Music can also help block out the little voice in your brain telling you it's time to quit. Research shows that this dissociation effect results in a 10 percent reduction in perceived effort during treadmill running at a moderate intensity.

PROMOTE SLEEP: Researchers have shown just 45 minutes of relaxing music before bedtime can make for a restful night. Taiwanese researchers studied the sleeping patterns of 60 elderly people with sleep problems. The study participants were either given a choice of music to listen to before going to sleep or nothing at all. Listening to music caused physical changes that aided restful sleep, including a lower heart and respiratory rate, the researchers found.

CONTROL APPETITE: Listening to music triggers an increase in the body's serotonin levels, and serotonin affects how much you feel like eating. When you have enough serotonin, you don't need to eat as much to feel full. On the other hand, when going into a meal with low serotonin, you'll have a tougher time sensing when your appetite is satisfied.

Find Yourself: Get Lost in a Book

According to a recent Pew Research Poll, fewer people are reading than ever before. In fact, 19 percent of respondents said they hadn't read a single book (either electronic or print) over the previous 12 months. Those who love books already know the joys of reading – how it enriches our inner lives, feeds our minds and imaginations, makes us happy, and offers us a sense of well-being. But did you know reading offers all these benefits, too?

RELIEVE STRESS: Removing oneself from a tense day by escaping into a fictional world has been shown to lower blood pressure and reduce stress. Say "good-bye" to stress binging.

IMPROVE CONCENTRATION: Following the printed word in a book requires focus for a longer period of concentration than reading e-mails, magazine articles, or web postings. This means less time focused on your appetite.

INCREASE VOCABULARY: Remember in elementary school when you learned how to infer the meaning of one word by reading the context of the other words in the sentence? You get the same benefit from book reading. Talk about a confidence-builder!

HEIGHTEN CREATIVITY: When you expose yourself to new ideas and information, your mind opens to fresh, creative avenues. When you're in the creative zone, the last thing you're likely to be thinking about is food.

SUPPORT SLEEP PATTERNS: If you make reading a habit before bed, a book acts as a kind of alarm for the body and sends the signal that it is time to sleep. Countless studies show sleeplessness is connected to weight gain.

BUILD SELF-ESTEEM: When we're better informed, we feel better about ourselves. Become an "expert" and people will come to you for answers. What an ego boost.

IMPROVE MEMORY: Studies show if you don't use your memory, you lose it. Reading helps you stretch your "memory muscles" in a similar way. Reading requires remembering details, facts, and figures and in literature that also means plot lines, themes, and characters. Ultimately, reading can boost your calorie-counting skills! Who knew?

ENHANCE DISCIPLINE: We all know we *should* read. Adding time to read a book as part of your daily schedule and sticking to it improves discipline. Discipline is a key to cleanse success.

CHANGE YOUR LIFE: Sometimes a book can be transformative and put you on a different path. You might decide to delve into a new hobby, pursue a different job, look at relationships differently, and decide to follow through on a health or fitness plan. That's the point about reading–it opens your world.

Embrace Your Artistic Side

Have you had the urge to follow your artistic instinct? But rather than pursue it, you've stifled the urge knowing you're far from a Picasso? Well, medical experts suggest we change our thinking. Research shows that making art (whether we're truly talented or not) not only boosts our brain power, but improves our overall well-being. Here's how:

PUT THE PRESENT IN FOCUS: Creating art means you have to pay attention to the here and now rather than daydreaming or getting caught in habitual thought loops. This kind of moment-to-moment presence eliminates distractive thinking.

STIMULATE IMAGINATION: If you've always considered yourself a left-brained person (practical, good with numbers, and analytical), you can change your mind. When you create art, it helps to awaken the right side of your brain to creativity and imagination and ultimately affects not only your artwork but how you see the world in general.

TWEAK SELF-ESTEEM: Remember how you used to put your kid's artwork on the fridge or walls? Now it's your turn. Hanging your latest work of art on the wall or displaying it on a shelf in your house instills the same feeling of pride and accomplishment.

SHARPEN ATTENTION: How often have you suddenly realized there's been a change on a familiar street and you hadn't noticed it? Well, Leonardo da Vinci said, "Painting embraces all the ten functions of the eye; that is to say, darkness, light, body and color, shape and location, distance and closeness, motion and rest." Creating art helps you to concentrate on detail and pay more attention to your environment – including your food.

HELP PROBLEM SOLVING: There are no correct answers in art. That's why art–making encourages creative, out–of–the box solution solving. Once you start using your creative brain, you'll be amazed at how differently you'll approach problems.

REDUCE STRESS AND DEPRESSION: Countless studies show pouring your attention into a soothing hobby like art bumps up your endorphins and reduces stress. It simply takes your mind off your worries and places them in a different part of your brain. FYI: Blood pressure can also drop.

Practice Loving Kindness

In a culture that prides itself on competition and individuality, sometimes loving kindness is put on the back burner. But compassion toward ourselves and others is a positive tool benefiting us both psychologically and physically. Open your heart and you'll *tame the stress response*: A study from Emory University concluded that compassionate meditation lessened inflammatory responses to stress, which in turn was a means of reducing depression, heart disease, diabetes, and weight gain.

MAKE CHANGING EASIER: Unsavory habits – whether its anger, laziness, procrastination, or junk food eating – tend to stick even harder when we identify them as parts of ourselves that we don't like. But studies show when we turn towards bad habits with loving kindness and understanding, they're easier to release.

RELEASE JUDGMENT: Are you Judge Judy? If you find yourself scrutinizing others harshly, there's a good chance your inner critic is also hard at work. Developing compassion and loving kindness releases both your inner and outer critic.

SECURE SELF-CONFIDENCE: Studies consistently show that those who rate highest on scales of self–esteem are also the most compassionate. It makes sense. Why does it make sense? Because in order to love and accept others, you need to feel the same way about yourself.

For all of us, love can be the natural state of our own being; naturally at peace, naturally connected, because this becomes the reflection of who we simply are."

~ *Sharon Salzberg*,
Loving Kindness, The
Revolutionary Art of
Happiness

7

How Far Have You Come?

Do you wake before the sunrise, like to read before bed, eat
on the go, finish your work right away – or procrastinate?
Everything in the universe is connected, and that's why every
choice you make and every habit you have is a clue to how
much you've gotten out of cleansing. Take this quiz to find out
what's hidden in your habits, how far you've come – and how
far you'll go!

Quiz
Rate Your Progress

1. You keep your house keys:
   a. On a table by the door.
   b. In your purse.
   c. Handy, in your pockets.

2. On weekends, you:

    a. Usually wake the same time as weekdays.

    b. Set your alarm for a couple of hours later.

    c. Try to rise by noon.

3. Your usual evening snack is:

    a. Fruit.

    b. Whatever tempts your taste buds.

    c. A hot drink.

4. You pay your bills:

    a. As soon as they arrive.

    b. On the first of the month.

    c. When you have the time.

5. Your bathing routine is:

    a. A speedy shower in the morning.

    b. Showering leisurely either morning or evening.

    c. Luxuriating in an evening bath.

6. Your desk or work area…

    a. Is organized with a place for pens, clips, etc.

    b. Neat with containers you've created.

    c. Has piles of paper everywhere…but you know where to find everything.

7. Your everyday bag is:

    a. Compact — just for essentials.

    b. A mid-size shoulder bag with room enough for a journal, book, or knitting.

    c. An extraroomy tote that holds everything.

8. You make a meal special:

    a. By sticking to the letter of a recipe.

    b. Tapping into your own inspiration all the way.

    c. Concentrating on what you're eating.

9. During a meeting you are usually:

   a. Taking notes.

   b. Doodling.

   c. Writing down ideas.

10. To go from floor to floor at a mall, if available, you would take the:

   a. Glass elevator.

   b. Escalator.

   c. Stairs.

11. Your daily to-do list is:

   a. All checked off! Done!

   b. Everything fun is done!

   c. Which to-do list?

Mostly A's: You're the Take-Charge Type

Clear–sighted, ultraorganized, and disciplined, your everyday habits include sticking to a to–do list, avoiding distractions, and thinking ahead, staying prioritized and super–focused. Plus, you never have to wait for motivation to get going! That's why you've been able to stick to the Superfood Cleanse without any difficulty and you'll continue to do so in the future. Thanks to your past successes, deep down you believe in yourself. You have an inner drive that leads you to face obstacles head on because you make it a habit to take decisive, positive action. Even the occasional slip doesn't get you down. It only fuels your determination to do better on the next cleanse day.

Mostly B's: You're a Creative Dynamo

Vision and passion fuel your habits, so you pursue only what feeds your inspiration. It's common for you to think outside the box. That's why your daily life is filled with spontaneous decisions and unique choices. While friends opt for a trip to the mall, you might be more in the mood to curl up on the couch and write in your journal. Who knows? You've got the spirit of a true artist! As your habits show, you may not take the straight and narrow, and that's why you have a tougher time sticking to an eating regimen, but you always make your life a beautiful creation – moment to moment. Forgive yourself for slipups and then get back on track.

Mostly C's: You're the Consummate Juggler

A master at multitasking, you can change direction on a dime. No wonder you always get a ton done. Your daily habits show you've learned to transition from one task to the next while staying focused and tuning out distractions. An excellent time keeper, you're also able to intuitively know what's most crucial and take care of the pressing problems before moving to the next task. Experts say this kind of "helicopter view" allows you to stay clear and flexible because you always see the big picture. But you're also a victim of stress, which may trigger less healthy food choices. Be aware of when you need downtime to rejuvenate. Use the tips on developing a healthy inner life to help you relax.

Final Thoughts for a Successful Superfood Cleanse

GIVE YOURSELF TIME: Whenever you have the urge to opt out of the cleanse, wait another 15 to 30 minutes. Studies show this habit will help you stay the course.

SUBSTITUTE A BAD HABIT WITH A GOOD ONE: Schedule in "guilt-free play time" each week. This will help cancel out bad habits and double your effectiveness and joy!

PAY THE CONSEQUENCES: If you don't stick with the cleanse, pay a fine, whether it's cleaning a friend's house or cutting out dessert on non-cleanse days. Consequences help boost willpower. Conversely, when you achieve a goal, reward yourself!

Yesterday is gone. Tomorrow has not yet come. We have only today. Let us begin.

~ Mother Teresa

Conversions

Common Conversions

1 gallon = 4 quarts = 8 pints = 16 cups = 128 fluid ounces = 3.8 liters
1 quart = 2 pints = 4 cups = 32 ounces = .95 liter
1 pint = 2 cups = 16 ounces = 480 ml
1 cup = 8 ounces = 240 ml
¼ cup = 4 tablespoons = 12 teaspoons = 2 ounces = 60 ml
1 tablespoon = 3 teaspoons = ½ fluid ounce = 15 ml

Temperature Conversions

Fahrenheit (°F)	Celsius (°C)
200°F	95°C
225°F	110°C
250°F	120°C
275°F	135°C
300°F	150°C
325°F	165°C
350°F	175°C
375°F	190°C
400°F	200°C
425°F	220°C
450°F	230°C
475°F	245°C

Volume Conversions

U.S.	U.S. equivalent	Metric
1 teaspoon	½ fluid ounce	15 milliliters
1 tablespoon	2 fluid ounces	60 milliliters
1 cup	3 fluid ounces	90 milliliters
1 pint	4 fluid ounces	120 milliliters
1 quart	5 fluid ounces	150 milliliters
1 liter	6 fluid ounces	180 milliliters
1 ounce (dry)	8 fluid ounces	240 milliliters
1 pound	16 fluid ounces	480 milliliters

Weight Conversions

U.S.	Metric
½ ounce	15 grams
1 ounce	30 grams
2 ounces	60 grams
¼ pound	115 grams
1/3 pound	150 grams
½ pound	225 grams
¾ pound	350 grams
1 pound	450 grams

Index

About the Author

Robin Westen received an Emmy Award for the ABC health show *FYI*. She is currently the medical director for Thirdage.com, the largest health site for baby boomers on the Web. She is the author of *The Yoga-Body Cleanse* and *Ten Days to Detox, the Harvard Medical School Guide Getting Your Child to Eat (Almost) Anything*, as well as *V is for Vagina*, which is coauthored with Alyssa Dweck, MD. She's written feature articles for dozens of national magazines including *Glamour, Vegetarian Times, Psychology Today, SELF, Cosmopolitan*, and others. Robin has been practicing yoga, meditation, and cleansing for over fifteen years. She divides her time between Brooklyn and Vermont.